WHAT THE STARS & EXPERTS SAY ABOUT THIS BOOK!!!

"Follow this book and your children will be faster than a speeding bullet, be able to leap tall buildings with a single bound, and wipe up the floor with you by the time they're nine."

Danny DeVito & Rhea Perlman

"This is the first and best book we've ever read on family nutrition ...the recipes are delicious!"

Lisë & Mac Davis

"Our children have grown to be as strong and healthy as they are in large part (due to) Dr. Gordon's presence in their lives. His commitment to their well-being and sound nutrition has been an inspiration to us."

Mel Harris ("Hope" on *thirtysomething*)
and Cotter Smith

"With the support, guidance, and expertise of Dr. Gordon....we feel 100% confident and excited in raising our children with these new invaluable guidelines."

Deborah & Olympic Gold Medalist Mitch Gaylord

"Jay is a physician for all seasons...it takes a true healer to encourage us to find that place of wellness and self-reliance where healing is no longer needed."

Michael Ontkean

"This is the first book to correctly address the nutritional needs of children. The information could be life saving."

.D.
am

i

"Good Food Today, Great Kids Tomorrow is one of the most valuable gifts parents can give to their children. . . a lifetime of healthy habits, good eating, and happiness."

Keenen Ivory Wayans
Executive Producer, "In Living Color"

"(We) are so grateful for your book. We have struggled with food allergies for years with our children, and have found that the only way to eat is exactly what you endorse."

Linda Kelsey
actress in *Lou Grant*

"Jay Gordon has cared for our children. He asks, "do you eat your vegetables?" "Yes!", my kids say with glee. "Do we eat candy all day?!" "No!" . . . So goes a check-up with pediatrician Jay Gordon. . . Dr. Gordon has not removed all the trials and tribulations for parents from childrearing, but he has made a start."

Melissa Mathison Ford
(Mrs. Harrison
Ford)

"Dr Jay has been our son's pediatrician since day one. We love his advice, value his judgment, and Sam eats his vegetables!!"

Michael J. Fox & Tracy Pollan

"If you want healthy children with controlled weight and increased longevity, then add Jay Gordon's book to your family medical library. This is a wake-up call to all parents!"

Dan and Donna Aykroyd

ii

Good Food Today
Great Kids Tomorrow

50 Things You Can Do
For Healthy, Happy Children

Jay Gordon, M.D.

with
Antonia Barnes Boyle

Published by Michael Wiese Productions, 11288 Ventura Blvd., Suite 821, Studio City, California, 91604, (818) 379-8799

Cover Design by Chris Whorf, The Art Hotel, Los Angeles
Author photograph by Geraldine Overton
Illustrations by Rick Stromoski

Printed by Braun-Brumfield, Inc., Ann Arbor, Michigan
Manufactured in the United States of America
Copyright 1994 by Jay Gordon, M.D.
First Printing September 1994

Printed on Recycled Paper

Gordon, Jay, 1948-

   Good food today, great kids tomorrow : 50 things you can do for healthy, happy children / by Jay Gordon, with Antonia Barnes Boyle.
       p.   cm.
ISBN 0-941188-17-5
1. Children -- Nutrition. 2. Vegetarian children. I. Boyle, Antonia Barnes, 1939- . II. Title.
Rj206.G58   1994
613.2'083--dc20   94-6672
                                                     CIP

TABLE OF CONTENTS

TABLE OF CONTENTS

ACKNOWLEDGMENTS

To my wife, Meyera Robbins, who first showed me that healthy food actually tastes much better than unhealthy food. I could not have done this without her help. She has encouraged me, coached me, inspired me, and occasionally, pushed me to write this book and get it done on time...or almost on time.

Meyera has somehow found the time to gather hundreds of recipes and tips which will make the programs I outline come alive for you: it really <u>is</u> much more fun and interesting to prepare healthy, good-tasting food for our children and families.

As I worked on this book, I called upon my office staff to find facts that were hidden, phone numbers I'd forgotten, and to coordinate meetings in a schedule filled to the brim already. They did all this and more. Lisa Boehle, Susan Whiteside, and Ileana Hernandez did a ton of extra work for me and the rest of my wonderful staff supported them and covered for them while they were absorbed with my requests.

Michael Wiese, my publisher, convinced me that I could do this even though I had made dozens of false starts in the past. He sat with me and asked me question after question to draw out the heart of this book. He then found Toni Boyle to work with me and shape my thoughts and ideas into coherence. Ken Lee, Michael's associate, made a never-ending stream of phone calls to keep me on track and on time. Robin Quinn, a copy editor with an uncanny eye for detail, did a terrific job cleaning up my initial draft for the book.

When the book was almost finished, I called upon the person I trust the most to critique not just the syntax and editing, but the feeling of the book: my sister, Jan Gordon. She helped put the book into its finished state.

I have learned more about realistic nutritional goals from the children and parents in my practice than from any book or mentor. When it came time to sit down and talk some more, these same people generously offered even more help. A very special thanks to these valued friends.

INTRODUCTION

INTRODUCTION

I am a doctor who specializes in the care of children. Every year, I see hundreds of youngsters from birth to college age. I watch out for their health needs. I make notes on when infants begin to nurse, and when children first eat solid foods. I listen to the parents who come to me more than occasionally confused, perplexed over the changes in their children, demonstrating a desire to give their youngsters the best possible foundation for the future. I have taken young patients through the traumas of nursery school and the elementary grades. I've done high school physical exams and filled out college health forms.

What all this has taught me is that there is a distinct and crucial relationship between the way children eat and how healthy they are. The parents of my patients are made aware of my views on nutrition, and I never have a child in my office for a check-up without talking about what foods they consume. When a child turns three, I begin to talk to them directly during each visit about how best to build strong bodies by eating only the best foods. The children become involved in the process of choosing a diet that's nutritious and promotes good health.

In this book, you will learn about the new list of basic food groups: fruits, vegetables, legumes, and grains. These foods should make up your child's entire diet. What I recommend in this book is a vegetarian or nearly vegetarian approach to eating. That's right – I believe that beef, fish, and poultry don't belong on your shopping list. As you read further, you'll learn why.

As you proceed through this book, you'll discover that the sugar your child eats should come naturally from fresh fruits. You'll learn that the fats in their diet should be reduced to very small amounts.

At first, this way of eating may be very different from your present routine, but I want to give your children and your family the very best diet plan available. If you follow it closely and lovingly for your children (and I know you can!) they will receive the benefits of growing sturdy bones, having fewer illnesses, and being less allergic to various foods. Your children will be able to pay attention better in school and play longer and harder.

It is a tragic fact that the majority of children six years and older exhibit the beginnings of fatty deposits in their arteries. This information comes from autopsy reports from child accident victims. In the 1950's, a vast majority of the young American casualties of the Korean war showed significant narrowing of the coronary arteries. This was during a time when there was less information available about eating low-fat foods. Like these young soldiers, many of our pre-teen and teenagers are on their way to life-shortening heart disease!

Every meal you feed your child from his birth on can lead him to heart disease. Or, on the correct diet – the one I'll outline on these pages – heart disease caused by fatty plaque collecting in the arteries does not have to be a threat at any age. The choice is up to you!

For most of you, the diet I've outlined is far different from the food that was served at the dinner table when you were growing up. It's a so-called *new* way of eating that is as old as our planet.

I believe that because of our physical make-up, we are meant to eat a meat-free, low-fat diet. Research by Dr. T. Colin Campbell of Cornell University in upstate New York has shown that the more vegetarian a diet is the healthier it is. Campbell, a nutritional biochemist, has studied the relationship between diet and disease for over 30 years. In a continuous

4

study which started in 1983 involving thousands of subjects in China, he has found that a vegetarian diet helps build a resistance to chronic, degenerative diseases such as cancer and heart disease.

Vegetarians include many people whose names you'd recognize. A list compiled for the February 1994 issue of *Vegetarian Times* includes some individuals you might expect and others that will surprise you. Steve Martin, Paul and Linda McCartney, Rosanna Arquette, Danny Glover, Christie Brinkley, Fred Rogers from Mr. Rogers, Marilu Henner, Dustin Hoffman, William Shatner, Casey Kasem from "American Top 40," Toni Tenille from Captain & Tenille, Hank Aaron, Sara Gilbert, Bryan Adams, Kim Basinger, body builder Andreas Cahling, Jerry Garcia of the Grateful Dead, and U.S. Congressman Andrew Jacobs from Indiana all made the magazine's "Celebrity Round-up" of known vegetarians.

Our bodies need fruits and vegetables, and the full range of rices, cereals, beans, and pastas that are available. The variety of foods on this plan is almost limitless. After some adjustment, I think you'll find a vegetarian or nearly vegetarian diet to be a comfortable, easy, healthy, and very tasty way to eat.

In addition to being a pediatrician, I'm also a father. Parenting my daughter, Simone, has added a dimension to my life that's quite apart from any medical training I've received. My main goal in life is to give Simone the optimal chance for a healthy lifetime. That's why Simone eats the diet I recommend in this book. She's a strong, seven-year-old, life-long vegetarian. She doesn't eat meat, poultry, or fish. She enjoys a treat of frozen yogurt – too often, I sometimes think – but I've learned to relax as I see how healthy the rest of her diet remains. She eats little fat or sugar. She loves a crunchy apple or a handful of grapes, and she eats enormous amounts of fruits and pasta.

Is she deprived? Definitely not! She is bright, alert, happy, and fun-loving. She embodies all the traits that a parent or a pediatrician could hope for in a child. I want that same vibrant health for your children and for all youngsters. Without reservation, I believe in the easy, healthy diet I will explain in the following pages – even though it may seem to you to be a drastic departure from the way your parents taught you to eat. In *Good Food Today, Great Kids Tomorrow*, I'll explain in detail how this diet will benefit your children. You'll be given methods for changing from the far-from-healthy, American diet to a much healthier, high-fruit, high-vegetable, high-grain lifestyle in a two-week period. You'll learn how to restock your pantry and cook old traditional, favorite dishes in new ways.

This is an exciting step for you to take – a step towards enhanced wellness. You probably have some important questions about the changes you're about to consider. As you read these pages, you'll find answers to the questions my patients have asked me as they've made these critical changes to their family's diet. I've seen this diet work for my patients hundreds of times and in my own home for many years. I want you to see it work in **your** home, too.

PART ONE
DEFINING HEALTHY FOODS

DEFINING HEALTHY FOODS

One of the questions I hear most often concerns the definition of "healthy." Like every parent, you want to be certain
your child is as healthy as possible. In this section, we'll talk
about what that entails and the steps you can take today to
ensure your child's continuing health in the future.

1. *Everything I read has a different definition of "healthy." How
do I know if my children are healthy?*

I can understand your frustration. As we learn more and
more about our bodies, it becomes increasingly difficult to sort
out facts from fallacies. Let me put things in perspective for you.

A healthy child is not just free of disease; he also functions
at his best throughout the day. He plays hard, concentrates easily, has good stamina, and a pleasant disposition. He rarely
complains of stomach aches, and he sleeps well. In my clinical
experience, this is also a child who is eating the right foods.
He avoids fats and sugars while eating lots of fiber. The best
sources of fiber are legumes (dried beans and peas) (See
Glossary, p. 209) grains, fresh fruits, and vegetables.

When I try to talk to my young patients about this, they
take great delight in telling me about all the people they know
who eat junk food and are "doing fine." That's when I explain
that if you build a wall out of crumbly bricks and use library
paste for mortar, it might look like a great wall for a short time.
However, when it's 20 or 30 years old, that wall is going to
start crumbling. In the same way, bones and muscles that are
built out of junk food aren't going to last as long as those built
out of the best food available.

During the first few years of your child's life, you are in complete charge of what he eats and drinks. There is no excuse for not guiding him through those formative years with an excellent diet. You'll be establishing patterns which will last the next 80 years or more. It's one of the best gifts you'll ever give your child: good health and good eating habits.

2. *I want only the best for my child, but I don't want to take away his choices. How can I lead him toward the highest level of health possible?*

The optimal way for children and adults to eat is to center their diet around fruits, vegetables, legumes, and grains. Legumes, which include all the dried beans such as garbanzos, lentils, lima beans, split peas, kidney beans, and so on, are the highest source of vegetable protein. All the fresh vegetables and fruits give you vitamins and minerals. The grains, such as brown rice, millet, buckwheat, and amaranth provide protein and fiber.

When these foods make up your diet, you're on an optimal plateau. When you choose to add meat, fish, or dairy to your diet, you may lessen the benefits of a proper diet. The way most people eat today is a radical departure from what will promote good health.

I'm not trying to tell you that you can't have a special treat now and then. There will always be special occasions. A family birthday or holiday party is a time when you may want to indulge yourself and your children. The occasional deviation from your healthy eating plan isn't going to ruin your health. The danger is that you begin to think that one slip didn't hurt so two or three slips won't hurt either. This can lead to establishing new unhealthy habits that snap back at you later.

9

Children can be kept on an optimal food plan for several years without much effort. Up to the age of three or so, you simply tell the child, "We don't have any cookies in the house. We don't eat candy. Our family doesn't eat meat." Children during these years will eat what is fed to them.

Around age three, you will probably have to do more explaining. This is when you can begin to talk about growing strong muscles so they can run fast and play hard. When they're old enough to go to parties and preschool, they'll become aware of other food choices. That is the time to explain why they must continue to eat the way they've been taught at home.

I agree that children must learn to make their own choices. But if those choices involved crossing the street or playing with matches, you'd quickly take the right to choose out of their hands. To my mind, allowing a child to select unhealthy foods is just as dangerous.

Young children don't think of the long-term effects of an action. For that matter, neither do teenagers. That's why it's so important to instill proper eating habits into your children early so proper food choices are second nature by the time they are ready for high school.

Usually when a parent comes into my office with a child suffering from an intestinal disturbance, they already know about the "BRAT Diet." The letters are an acronym for Bananas, Rice, Apples, and Tea – the traditional foods used to soothe intestinal discomfort. I modify the BRAT Diet to include toast instead of tea, and tell parents to use it while serving no protein to children with intestinal disturbance.

Instead of just making the BRAT diet a remedy, parents can make it the healthy foundation of their children's daily diet. I suggest they add in other fruit and grains and a variety of other vegetables. This is food you can give a child not only while he's sick but every day for the rest of his life. This is the diet that promotes both healing and optimum health!

10

PART TWO
DANGEROUS FOODS

DANGEROUS FOODS

The old theories about which foods are best for growing children have been debunked in recent years. The basic food groups have been restructured dramatically. In this section, you'll discover why some of the foods that have long been considered essential building blocks for young bodies are, in reality, among the most detrimental to your child's health.

3. *Doesn't my daughter need milk and other dairy products so she can grow strong bones and teeth?*

Thanks in part to lobbying efforts on behalf of dairy farmers, Americans feel that it's necessary to drink milk throughout their lives. We've seen countless advertisements which perpetuate the myth: "Milk. It does a body good." Milk can be a high fat product with excessive quantities of protein. It's specifically designed to efficiently grow a cow, an animal which will mature rapidly and live a relatively short time. The National Research Council, a nonprofit organization that provides scientific advice to the federal government, has reported that the cow's milk humans drink also contains all of the pesticides and hormones that cows ingest with the alfalfa they eat.

A study published in the "American Journal of Clinical Nutrition" in June, 1993, confirmed that there is a definite correlation between cow's milk and the incidence of diabetes. Furthermore, some allergies which manifest themselves in runny and stuffy noses can be traced to cow's milk. Some ear and tonsil infections also originate with the drinking of milk. Ingesting other dairy products including butter, cheese, and ice cream can also result in these symptoms.

13

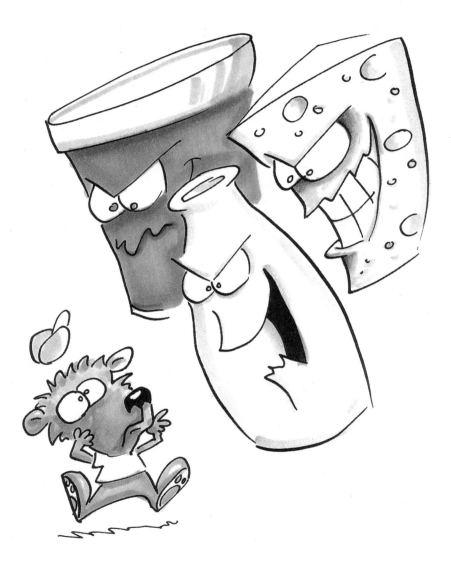

14

Surprisingly, we are the only species on this planet that drinks milk after infancy, and we are also the only species that drinks milk from a species other than our own. Maybe the other animals know more than we do!

Many infants have trouble digesting cow's milk. This intolerance of lactose (see Glossary, page 209, or to the protein in milk, manifests itself in stomach and intestinal disturbances, gas, and rashes.

Lactose is the result of combining two sugars: glucose and galactose. Most of us produce an intestinal enzyme, lactase, which allows us to break down these sugars. Our bodies produce the most lactase (see Glossary, page 209) in infancy when we drink the most milk. As we get older, our bodies produce lesser amounts of lactase so our tolerance to lactose goes down naturally.

The protein we get from milk can be obtained from dozens of vegetable sources, primarily legumes which include soy bean products. It is a little trickier to find other sources of calcium but this substance is contained in many vegetables like broccoli. Calcium is also available, in smaller amounts, in many other foods. If you're still concerned, you can buy calcium supplements wherever vitamins are sold. Soy milk, orange juice, and cereals are now calcium fortified.

I want you to be aware that cow's milk can show up in unexpected food items so you have to read labels carefully. Even a small amount hidden in a food can trigger a reaction in children with milk protein allergies.

I heard butter is better for you than margarine. Is this true?

No, definitely not! In fact, in my opinion, butter may be the worst dairy product of all. It's nothing but congealed grease. Since it's the fattiest part of milk, it carries the most pollutants. This is because many pollutants are fat-loving, fat-soluble chemicals. It can also directly contribute to a dramatic increase in heart disease, a condition which begins in the first five years of a child's life even though it may not kill until many years later. I don't think children or anyone, for that matter, should eat butter.

Let's be very clear about another popular misconception. Margarine isn't any better than butter. Even though it's a vegetable product, margarine is greasy and full of "trans fats" (see Glossary on page 211). Trans fats, which are liquid vegetable oils that have been hydrogenated (see Glossary on page 209) to make them spreadable and to increase their stability, have been proven to increase the incidence of cancer. A study by the Harvard School of Public Health states that margarine is associated with a 70% increase in the risk of heart disease in women. Dr. Walter Willet, who authored a study published in a British medical journal, *Lancet*, in March, 1993, advocates the use of soybean, corn, or canola oil to replace the partially hydrogenated vegetable fats found in most margarine.

Researchers have found that when women eat four or more teaspoons of margarine a day, they are at significantly greater risk for heart disease than women who eat two teaspoons or less during the same period. Furthermore, they have discovered that this increased risk is also present when the hydrogenated vegetable fats are consumed in breads and cookies.

Be safe! Stay away from butter and margarine and the processed foods that contain them. You and your children will be healthier without them!

My son loves cheese. Is it safe to give him a little?

I believe that eating cheese is worse than eating candy. I view it as the ultimate junk food. In fact, so-called "low-fat" cheese has one of the highest fat contents of anything in the supermarket! When your child gets a piece of cheese, you're handing him the type of food that can ultimately close his arteries and increase his chances of getting intestinal cancer. In females, animal fat is indisputably linked to cancer of the cervix and breast.

While there are no-fat cheeses on the market now, they are often very bland. And, unfortunately, cheese made from soybean milk, like margarine, is one of a few vegetable products that's very high in fat and salt.

I strongly recommend that you take cheese out of your diet. I want to make this point very clear. All cheese is made from milk. It can promote allergic reactions. It can begin the closure of the arteries due to the build-up of plaque. It has been related to the growth of colon tumors. Think of the health problems promoted by these chunks of flavored fat! I don't advocate serving cheese to anyone.

The Truth about "Low-Fat" Cheese

Low fat cheeses are very popular, and we see more and more of them in the supermarkets. At first glance, the low-fat cheeses seem like a good answer. But if you compare the labels of a whole-milk cheese and its low fat knock-off, you'll notice some disturbing facts.

Let's take mozzarella, as an example. Three and a half ounces of whole-milk mozzarella has 318 calories and 25 grams of fat (16 grams of which are saturated). It also contains 415 mg of sodium. The same amount of low fat cheese, its supposedly healthier cousin (made with skim milk), has 280 calories, 17 grams of fat (11 grams of which are saturated), and a whopping 528 mg of sodium. That's a lot of calories, fat, and sodium for 3 1/2 ounces of food!

My recommendation is: "Don't eat cheese – whether it's the regular or the low-fat variety!"

I understand about butter and cheese, but you can't mean that a scoop of ice cream is going to do any harm?

Ice cream has all the bad properties we've talked about in the other dairy products. It's full of fats and contains all the pollutants found in milk. It also packs the added whammy of being full of sugar. Ice cream clogs your children's arteries, slows down their energy level, and makes them fat. If only for the sake of your child's self-esteem, keep her away from food that can contribute to being overweight. I'd rather be trapped in a cage with hungry weasels than be in a second grade classroom with other kids who thought I was fat. No ice cream cone in the world is worth it.

Frozen yogurt is a little less damaging, but it's no bargain. The main problem with frozen yogurt is that it is a dairy product which contains sugar or some other type of sweetener. I have young patients with recurrent ear infections who have been cured by taking them completely off dairy. The best thing to do is to keep frozen bananas, strawberries, or raspberries in the freezer all the time and run them through a food processor when your child asks for something sweet to eat. Kids find it to be very tasty, and it's a harmless snack.

4.   *My toddler's favorite snack food is a couple of cocktail wieners. Should I let him have them?*

No. I consider hot dogs to be some of the scariest food around. They can be stuffed with unpleasant things, like chicken lips, pig's ears, and cow's innards. If the manufacturer's can't find anything else to do with the animal part, they grind it up, add lots of salt and fat for flavor, and stuff it in a hot dog casing. In hot dogs, Americans will eat food they'd never touch if they saw it in its original state.

Another danger of hot dogs is that every year a number of child deaths are reported because a piece of hot dog gets struck in the windpipe. Their size and shape make wieners dangerous to feed to a baby or toddler. Furthermore, I don't recommend them for children or adults because they contain both nitrates and nitrites (see Glossary, page 210). Both nitrates and nitrites have been shown to promote cancer.

How about hamburgers? I make sure I only buy ground round to get less fat and then I barbecue instead of frying.

Where do I start? Most often, hamburgers are made from less marketable cuts of meat which are high in fat. The 1993 E coli 0157:H7 bacteria scare, which involved the deaths of children due to undercooked hamburger, points to another reason to stay away from this food. When meat is taken from the dead animal carcass, it is often contaminated by excrement which contains the deadly E coli 0157:H7 strain of bacteria. In most cuts, the contamination remains on the top of the meat and is killed in the cooking process. (No matter how raw you want your steak, the surface is going to be well-cooked.) In hamburger, however, the contamination can be spread throughout the meat and may hide in the very center. If the patty isn't thoroughly cooked to precision temperature levels of at least 160 to 170 degrees, there is a chance that the cooked hamburger will harbor this E coli bacteria. Ingesting the bacteria can cause you or your child to get very sick or even die.

Furthermore, by barbecuing the meat, you're adding carcinogens which can lead to the development of cancer.

5. Our family doesn't eat any red meat. Isn't it healthier to stick to chicken and fish for our protein?

In America, chickens are raised in "poultry factories" where they are crowded together without enough space to move. This breeding system prevents the birds from running, and this ensures that their meat will be tender instead of tough and stringy. Because the birds are bred in such close proximity, they have to be medicated to guard against the diseases that are a natural product of living so near one another. They also receive chemicals to speed their growth so they can go to market heavier and sooner.

The lack of movement that breeds disease and stunts growth also causes the birds to become fat. Many cuts of chicken are much fatter than people realize. The average chicken leg without the skin is 30% fat and a thigh without the skin is 46% fat. Add the skin and a cooked leg will be 46% fat! A thigh cooked with skin is 56% fat! Try boiling a chicken in a pot and see how much fat rises to the top!

As long as we're talking about chickens, maybe I should say something about eggs. Here again, I advise that you remove them from your diet entirely. The yolks are full of fat and cholesterol. A typical egg yolk is a whopping 76% fat and contains 213 milligrams of cholesterol. Just take the yolk out of a hard-boiled egg and rub it between your fingers. You'll feel the grease. The white of the egg doesn't have the fat and cholesterol. Egg whites, however, not only can contain many contaminants from chicken feed, but they also can cause allergic reactions. The only part of an egg that I can say anything good about is the shell. It's not edible, of course, but at least it has a little calcium. Just skip eggs!

Fish is another food that I advise my patients not to eat. Many fish are high in fat. I'll give you a few examples: swordfish is 29.7% fat; shark, 30.8% fat; orange roughy, 50.4% fat; and atlantic salmon, 40.1% fat. (All of these fat assessments were made for fish in a raw state.) Cream-based sauces and butter sautéing can add even more fat to the fish dishes you eat! But even the lower fat fish, such as flounder (11.7% fat, cooked), halibut (18.9% fat, cooked), and sea bass (18.6%, raw), generate other health concerns.

Think about where fish live. Everything from human waste to industrial waste is poured into our rivers, lakes, and oceans. It is very difficult to find a piece of fish that hasn't been exposed to some contamination. The risks from eating contaminated fish include gastrointestinal illness and hepatitis.

Fresh water fish when cooked may be loaded with mercury, lead, and industrial pollutants like PCBs (Poly-Chlorinated Biphenyls) which are carcinogenic (see Glossary, page 206). Ocean fish can be equally contaminated. A number of studies have found swordfish to contain unhealthy levels of mercury. One study showed 43% of salmon tested had significant levels of PCBs.

Another concern is the lack of mandatory inspection for fish. When Consumers Union studied samples from fish bought at retail, it found that 29% were spoiled and almost 50% were contaminated with fecal bacteria. Additional toxins were found in another 44% of the fish tested.

In 1993, pregnant women, infants, and children were advised by the National Fisheries Institute to limit their consumption of swordfish and shark to once a month. This is because the U.S. Food and Drug Administration reported finding illegal levels of methyl mercury in one out of five samples of these types of fish during a three-year review. This should tell you something!

As far as I am concerned, fish and chicken aren't the best choices for sources of protein. They aren't necessarily low fat, and they pose other health concerns.

6.   *I hear a lot about "junk foods," but I'm not always sure what's included in that definition.*

Junk foods aren't just candy, potato chips, cookies, crackers, soft drinks, and French fries. They're also processed and over-processed foods found in the supermarket, often wrapped in cellophane. When you read the labels, you find that salt and sugar are high on the list of ingredients. Even a jar of spaghetti sauce may qualify as a junk food if it's high in oil, salt, and preservatives.

I encourage you to make every effort to serve whole foods (foods as they appear in nature), such as fresh vegetables, fruits, and grains. Whole foods that haven't had the vitamins and nutrients processed out of them are much better for you than TV dinners and potato chips.

This is a good time to mention those very common junk foods, soft drinks. It's hard to walk more than a few steps without bumping into someone who has a cola can in their hand. The truth is that soft drinks are nothing but gassy, flavored sugar water. To make things worse, they don't even quench thirst because the body loses liquid trying to digest the sugar. Furthermore, these drinks contain phosphoric acid which robs the body of calcium and is caustic enough to clean metal!

The one calorie variety are no better and, in some ways, may be even worse for you. Artificial sweeteners were never intended to be ingested in the large amounts we find in our foods today. I would rather a child have a little sugar than an artificial sweetener.

So soft drinks really do rate as liquid junk foods. They contain unhealthy amounts of sugar or sweetener, phosphoric acid, and gas. They offer only very low levels of nutrients and can actually make you thirstier. Keep them out of your child!

Instead of soft drinks, offer interesting fruit or vegetable juice combinations. Whenever possible, use your kitchen juicer and encourage your children to help you think up new ways to combine fruits. Always dilute fruit juices with an equal amount of water. For a special treat, you can add naturally-sparking mineral water. The 50-50 dilution of the juice with water will cut down on the amount of natural sugar your children get from the fruit. If you allow youngsters to drink pure fruit juice, you'll be very aware of the roller coaster effect sugar has on their emotions and behavior.

One more warning. If you read the labels, most fruit juice has words like "cocktail" or "flavored" on the label. These juices have a high concentration of sugar syrup. Always look for natural juices and make certain that you dilute them just as you do the fresh juice.

Where your children are concerned, water or diluted natural fruit juice is always a better choice.

Soft Drink Experiment

A convincing experiment for most children is to pour a glass of the most popular cola drink and leave a dirty penny in it overnight. The next morning, the penny will be as shiny as new. If cola does that to medal, think what it does to the lining of your child's stomach!

23

7.   I'm so grateful for artificial sweeteners. Aren't they a better way to give my children sweets without worrying about their reaction to sugar?

Artificial sweeteners were invented for one specific purpose: to provide sugar taste for medically supervised diabetics and dieters. No one could have foreseen the day would come when chemical sweeteners were in large percentage of the products we would eat every day. For instance, aspartame, which is marketed today under the trade names Equal® and NutraSweet®, was never intended to be ingested by children and adults all day long. In the 1990s, aspartame is found in most foods which are marked "Sugar-Free," from gelatin desserts and puddings to soft drinks and candies.

Aspartame is made by combining two amino acids. It is never to be taken by those who have PKU (phenylketonuria), an hereditary metabolic disorder (see Glossary, page 210). The FDA suggests that no more than 50 milligrams of aspartame per 2.2 pounds of body weight be consumed in any one day. For the average adult, this is about 17 cans of diet soda. For a 40-pound child, it translates to only four or five cans – assuming the sweetener is not in any other food eaten that day. With the prevalence of aspartame in the foods children consume, including packet fruit powders, gelatins, and puddings, it isn't difficult for a child to ingest more than the suggested amount in a 24-hour period.

In 1984, 3,341 tons of aspartame went into the foods Americans ate. Since aspartame is 180 times as sweet as sugar, that translates into the equivalent of 686,000 tons of sugar. By 1985, sales of the sweetener had already reached $700 million a year. Every year since then, artificial sweeteners have become a more significant component of processed foods. Why worry about possible adverse reactions? Simply stay away from artificial sweeteners.

Commercials try to promote these sweeteners as being safe because they are a harmless combination of naturally occurring elements. Ridiculous! Gunpowder is the combination of naturally occurring elements, and no one would presume for an instant that gunpowder is not dangerous. We don't have enough experience with the commercial sweeteners currently in our foods. We don't know if today's artificial sweeteners could have disastrous long-term consequences. An earlier sugar substitute, cyclamate, was found to promote cancer and was subsequently removed from the market in October 1969.

I see no reason why a child needs to be given sweetened food. There is plenty of sugar in the fruits that should be abundant in his diet. Even if, from infancy, he has never had sugar, you will find your child has a natural sweet tooth. If you don't believe this, try putting something sour on your baby's tongue and watch him make a "yucky face." Then try a little sugar. His face will relax, and you'll see the beginning of a smile. We are born with a "sweet tooth." The fact is that human breast milk is the sweetest produced by any mammal. You don't want to intensify your child's natural desire for sweets. So the secret is, as much as possible, to keep your children away from processed sugars and the foods that contain them.

8. *I only allow my child two pieces of candy a day. I don't have to refuse him that small pleasure, do I?*

You don't have to refuse your child a piece of candy – if it doesn't bother you that he's eating pure sugar at best and greasy sugar at worst. Candy provides virtually no nutritional benefits. I can't see that it has any place in a child's diet.

I always wonder when a parent tells me they don't know how to say "no" to a particular food. What if your toddler asked you for a glass of bourbon? I doubt you'd have any trouble refusing to allow it. Candy is in the same league. Because of the harm it can do to teeth, weight, and behavior, I view candy as a punishment instead of a treat.

We seem to have the most trouble refusing our children what we were refused at their age. The good news is that with practice "no" comes more easily.

In place of a piece of candy, offer a piece of fruit. It's also sweet and full of flavor, and contains 90% water which helps keep your child's hydration level high. Another benefit is, unlike candy, the fruit "wrapper" can go into the compost instead of the landfill.

PART THREE
HEALTHY FOODS

PART THREE: HEALTHY FOODS

Healthy foods are plentiful and provide abundant nutrition for your growing child. In this section, you will be introduced to organic foods, tofu, and the benefits of fat-free eating. You may be surprised to find out that peanut butter sandwiches should be a "no-no."

9. *What is the benefit of organic foods? Why should I spend extra money for them?*

Organic fruits and vegetables are raised by healthier methods, using no chemicals and pesticides. The problem with pesticides is that children, pound for pound, eat more bananas and drink more apple juice than adults. This means that if a certain amount of pesticide has been deemed safe for a 150 pound adult, it probably isn't safe for a 35 pound child. Very few adults drink apple juice or eat bananas with the fervor of toddlers. When children drink a quart of apple juice in a day and eat at least one banana, they're ingesting, pound for pound, more poison in their food during the years when they have the least tolerance.

Unfortunately, because less organic food is grown and marketed, the prices are somewhat higher. There was a time when you could only buy organically-grown foods in health food stores. Today, little by little, supermarkets are devoting a few precious feet of produce space to this important health product. We need to make ourselves heard at the grocery store. Where customers create a demand, product becomes available. Where product is readily available, costs come down.

Our daughter, Simone, was involved in a gardening project at her elementary school. The children were instructed on how to plant, tend, and harvest their own vegetables. The young-sters loved eating the vegetables they had raised, and they were proud of their efforts. You can get information on how to start such a program in your school by contacting the Outreach Coordinator for the Common Ground Garden Program, University of California Cooperative Extension for Los Angeles County, 2615 S. Grand Ave., #400, Los Angeles, CA 90007-2668. The telephone number is (213) 744-4349 and the FAX number is (213) 745-7513.

We've started a garden plot at home too. It's a wonderful way for me to become involved in the things that interest my daughter and, at the same time, teach her about what she should eat.

If you live in a city apartment, you can build your garden in pots on a windowsill or under fluorescent lights. Ask for guidance at your local garden center. There is nothing that compares with the taste of a tomato, warmed from the sun and picked by hand from your own garden.

10. *I keep hearing about "tofu." What is it and how do I use it?*

Tofu is a highly-versatile soy bean product, rich in protein and calcium. White and smooth, it comes in blocks and is a cross between a firm custard and soft cheese. You want to be very sure that the tofu you buy is made from organically-grown soybeans.

There are different consistencies of tofu – soft or silken and firm – depending on whether you want to use it as a dip or cut it into cubes to replace meat in stir fry and pasta dishes. Since it has almost no flavor of its own, tofu readily picks up the flavors of whatever is mixed with it. In the final section of this book, you'll find some delicious tofu recipes my wife Meyera, has created.

Cut as much fat as possible out of your children's diet. If they don't thank you now, they will later when they remain lean and healthy while their middle-aged friends are worrying about heart disease and spare tires.

Know Your Fats!

It's important to understand the different kinds of fat. The worst are called saturated fats (see Glossary, page 207), and are found in meat and dairy products as well as in coconut and palm oils. Monounsaturated fats (see Glossary, page 207, are the safest of the oils. We find monounsaturated fats in avocados and olives and their oils. The last category, polyunsaturated fats (see Glossary, page 208, include fish oils and most vegetable oils.

The unsaturated fats, especially polyunsaturated, are thought to lower total cholesterol. Hardening of the arteries may also be reduced. However, consumption of all fats should be kept low, and saturated fats in particular should be avoided.

Tofu is a medium calorie product (about 145 calories per 3 1/2 ounces), but it's fairly high in fat (about 9 grams per 3 1/2 ounces). It's an excellent source of protein and also supplies a good amount of calcium. The fat in tofu is mostly unsaturated, but 3 1/2 ounces almost uses up the daily fat allowance for an 1800 calorie diet that's typical for a three to ten-year-old child.

11. *Low-fat, no-fat, saturated fat – it's all very confusing. Don't children need fat during the early years?*

Most pediatricians agree that children need a significant amount of fat in their diet during the first two years of life. This is because the brain is developing and depends on a relatively high fat intake. During the time of brain development, the body is going through one of its most rapid growth periods. For instance, a typical child's head circumference will increase in size by three inches between birth and 12 months. It will then take 15 years to increase another three inches!

In the first 12 months, the average child will triple its birth weight and in the first four years of life, he or she will grow 20 inches.

Beyond the age of two or three, your child can be on a lowered fat diet. In cultures where childhood diets are high in fat and remain that way, the incidence of adult heart disease and cancer is significantly higher.

As parents, we give a gift to our children when we teach them that low fat food is tasty and preferable to butter, cheese, and ice cream. This doesn't mean you have to restrict or deprive your child of anything. It just means that you leave foods that can be harmful out of his diet! You'll find he feels better and behaves better when his meals are low in fat and consist predominantly of fruits, vegetables, and grains.

PART FOUR
THE SCIENCE OF FEEDING YOUR CHILDREN

THE SCIENCE OF FEEDING YOUR CHILDREN

Today people are more health and nutrition conscious than ever before in history. In this section, you will be introduced to the **Science of Feeding Your Child.** You will understand how protein is readily available when you're serving a meat-free diet and the role fiber, salt, and sugar play in your child's behavior patterns and optimum health.

12. If I don't feed my children meat, where are they going to get the protein they need?

There are two primary sources of protein, animals and plants. Plant sources include legumes and grains. The major concern with the avoidance of animal proteins has been the loss of complete amino acids. There are nine essential amino acids in meat protein, and no single plant product delivers a complete protein. However, by eating combinations of vegetables and grains, you can provide the equivalent protein that is found in meat. For instance, rice and beans eaten together, whole wheat bread with chick-pea spread (hummus), or even rice cakes with a spoonful of almond butter will provide as complete a protein as beef. It's not important that you eat all the essential amino acids in one meal. You can spread out your intake throughout the day.

It's important for you to understand how much protein we actually need: much **less** than most of us eat. On an average day, a child is given three times the amount of protein necessary for growth. The correct ratio is about one gram of protein per pound of body weight during the first year of life. This drops to about half a gram of protein per pound in the second through the fifteenth year. There are 28 grams to an ounce so we're not talking about very much in volume. If you weigh 135 pounds, you need only 2 1/2 ounces of protein a day!

Where do you get this protein? Right from your cupboards. Grains, cereals, pastas, tofu, and beans are all excellent sources of protein. As I've said, soybeans, from which tofu is made, provide the most complete of the plant proteins. A stir-fry meal made with tofu, instead of meat, and served on a bed of natural brown rice will provide plenty of good protein for children and adults.

Another good source of protein is a good, grainy pasta. Pasta dishes are universal favorites for children. Try making lasagna with tofu instead of ricotta cheese or stuff whole wheat pasta shells with spinach and tofu, cover them with a fresh tomato sauce, and bake the shells in the oven.

Legumes are another excellent source of protein. Meatless chili, hummus on pita bread, or almond butter on whole grain bread will supply your children with adequate protein as well as healthful fiber.

In any good bookstore, you can find booklets that will give you the protein, cholesterol, carbohydrate, fat, and sodium breakdowns of almost any food you could want to serve.

The list below shows the percentage of protein that each type of food contains. Here is a general guide to help you reach your nutritional goals for yourself and your family. Look to vegetables and grains as sources of carbohydrates. Legumes provide protein and carbohydrates. Nuts are a source of protein but usually contain so much fat that this outweighs the protein benefit. Meats and milk supply protein and fat. However, I am not recommending dairy or meat products.

PERCENTAGE OF PROTEIN CONTAINED

Vegetables

Brussels Sprouts	16%
Cabbage	17%
Carrots	10%
Corn	12%
Potatoes	11%
Tomatoes	16%

Grains

Bread(whole wheat)	16%
Brown Rice	8%
Oatmeal	16%
Spaghetti (whole wheat)	14%

Milk

Breast Milk	5%

Legumes/Nuts

Almonds	12%
Kidney Beans	26%
Peanuts	18%
Tofu (soy beans)	34%

Meats/Fish/Poultry

Beef	26%
Chicken	61%
Eggs	33%
Lobster	88%
Pork	42%
Turkey	68%

Cow's Milk	21%

13. *I've always heard that calcium is one of the building blocks of the body. Where is my child going to get calcium without dairy products?*

While calcium certainly is an essential building block for teeth and bones in a growing body, there is some dispute among medical professionals as to how much calcium we really need. The need for calcium is dependent on the increasing amount of protein a child takes in during the different growth phases. The Recommended Daily Allowance of calcium for an infant is 400 mg. a day for the first six months of life. This should be increased to 600 mg. a day for months six through 12. This need grows to 800 mg. for ages one through ten, and then jumps to 1200 mg. a day for ages ten through 18.

Dairy products have long been regarded as the easiest and the best source of calcium. However, the fats, allergic potential, and pesticide contaminants in milk make it an inappropriate source of calcium, in my opinion. I would never recommend that children drink four glasses of milk or eat yogurt every day. The thing you must understand is that there are other sources of calcium. They may be less convenient than opening the carton, but they are equally effective in supplying this needed mineral. Children who can't digest milk and dairy products grow well without them.

Broccoli, for instance, is an excellent source of calcium. It contains about the same amount as milk, ounce for ounce. Lightly steam and chill the flowerets so they're still a little crisp, and you'll have an excellent finger food that children will eat. You can even provide a little dish of fat-free salad dressing or yogurt that they can use for dipping. I recommend seven 1/2 cup servings a day of fruits and vegetables, balancing your choices from the two types of food. These seven servings will provide enough fiber, beta carotene, and vitamin C for any child.

Most of the dark green leafy vegetables provide calcium. The oxalic acid in spinach, however, actually retards the absorption of calcium. Spinach, of course, makes up for this minor deficiency by being an excellent source of iron.

If you have children who like kale, arugula, and dandelion greens, you'll have no trouble meeting their calcium requirements. Most of my young patients find those tastes too strong. You might try finely chopping the greens and adding them to a vegetable soup.

Sesame seeds are a good source of calcium, although they are high in fat. You can add sesame seeds to mashed potatoes or sprinkle them on salads. Sesame butter is available in health food stores. It can be used in place of peanut butter, which is very high in fat, sodium, and sugar when bought commercially. If your child demands peanut butter, use it only occasionally. Buy the natural variety which has no additives. Before using, allow the oil to flow to the top, and then pour it off before using the peanut butter.

As a final resort, especially if your child is going through a "picky eater stage," you can buy a liquid or chewable calcium supplement. If your child won't eat enough food during the day to satisfy you and his pediatrician that he's getting enough calcium, you can give supplements. Once a child is about three years old, you can give him 500 mg of chewable calcium. Balance this with about the same amount of magnesium. I suggest you put it into a blender drink, like a fruit smoothie, or into applesauce or mashed potatoes. That way you can be sure he's getting the amount he needs every day. If your child gets too much calcium on any particular day because of erratic eating habits, he will excrete the excess calcium.

14. *The whole question of vitamins is confusing. Do I need to give my twins vitamin supplements or will their food provide everything they need?*

I don't know a parent who isn't concerned about vitamins. The fact is there are vitamins in everything we eat. However, there is a connection between food, vitamins, and calories that is important to understand. For instance, when you eat a chunk of cheese, you get a lot of **calories per vitamin.** On the other hand, when you eat broccoli and cauliflower, you get a lot of **vitamins per calorie.** The better choice is obvious to me. I'd rather have my daughter eat a cup of vegetables to get her vitamins and, at the same time, she'll stay slim by avoiding all the fat in cheese.

In the best of all worlds, every child would eat a perfectly balanced diet to get just the right amount of vitamins. There was a time when we ate much differently. We would dig roots from earth that wasn't contaminated with pesticides and fertilizers. We'd pick fresh fruits and vegetables grown in soil that was still rich in nutrients. The diet that was adequate 50 years ago may no longer exist in this age of chemically-assisted agriculture and processed foods.

That's why I recommend supplemental vitamins after infancy. During the first year when children are breast-feeding or taking a formula, they are getting all the vitamins they need. After the ages of 12 to 18 months, I think it's a good idea to give a supplementary vitamin. Children who are going through growth spurts may temporarily outgrow their vitamin supply, and you can think of the supplemental vitamin as an insurance policy.

When choosing a supplemental multi-vitamin, go to a good health food store and find a formula without a lot of artificial colors or flavors. I like to recommend those which have large doses of the B vitamins, along with extra vitamin E, beta carotene, and large quantities of vitamin C. For younger children, a liquid vitamin is preferable to the chewable variety. Like other medicines, you can mix the vitamins in foods or drinks, and your child will take them without a fuss.

Vitamin B-6 & Folic Acid & Pregnancy

I'd like to point out a potential vitamin deficiency that every pregnant woman must understand. During pregnancy, it is necessary for the mother get the RDA of folacin and vitamin B-6. Also referred to as folic acid, folacin is essential for the production of genetic material in the cells and the formation of hemoglobin in red blood cells.

The lack of folic acid can cause the mother to become anemic and possibly miscarry. In the worst case scenario, the child may be born with a deformity.

Folacin is abundantly available in foods, including dark-green, leafy vegetables, fruits, and legumes. It is thought that the vitamin is lost when the foods are cooked so, as much as possible, eat the vegetables and fruits uncooked.

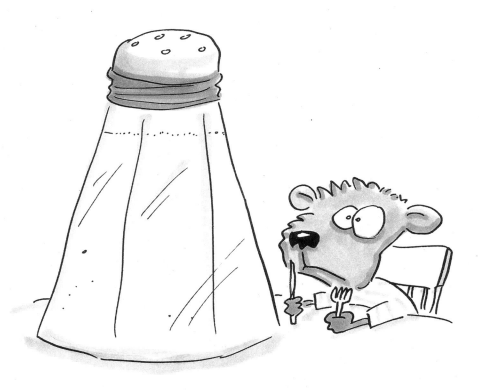

15. *My husband and I are both on sodium-restricted diets, so I never add salt to our food. Do our children need more salt in their diets?*

We *all* need a little salt in our diets. Sodium and chloride are essential nutrients. However, we get all the salt we need naturally in the foods we eat. There isn't any reason to add more salt when cooking or at the table.

When you have more salt than you need, you retain water in your tissues. The minerals in salt, combined with the water retention, raise your blood pressure. Even if you don't retain water in your tissues, it's known that salt has a definite adverse effect on your arteries. These physical reactions are most pronounced as you get older, but *the habits established in childhood influence the rest of your life!*

Unfortunately, we eat way too much salt. Processed foods have incredibly high sodium levels to mask the fact we've processed all the flavor out of the things we package. Fast food restaurants may give you double the daily recommended requirement of salt in just one order of a burger and fries or chicken nuggets. Chinese and Italian restaurants are no better according to reports from the Center for Science in the Public Interest in 1993 and 1994.

At home, read the labels on the food you serve your children, and you'll find that breakfast cereals may have as much sodium, ounce for ounce, as potato chips. Cheese is very high in sodium, as are deli meats, like turkey roll, ham, or bologna. The soy sauce that is used to enhance the flavor of Oriental food is almost pure salt. When you eat two slices of take-out pizza, you use up your full daily allotment of salt.

In our home, we use lemon and/or herbs in place of salt. Simone doesn't notice the difference. If your children are raised to enjoy the honest flavor of natural, unsalted foods, you'll be helping them be healthy while you train the taste buds to enjoy unsalted foods.

16. *I know cholesterol is dangerous for adults but children don't get hardening of the arteries, do they?*

Autopsies performed on children six year of age and older who have been killed in accidents have shown that the majority exhibit fatty streaks on their arteries along with some narrowing of the coronary arteries. An autopsy study conducted in the 1950's during the Korean War showed that 90 percent of the 20-year-old, American boys who were killed in battle had significant, if not critical, narrowing of some of the coronary arteries. This type of narrowing is caused by a diet high in fats and cholesterol.

Heart disease doesn't begin in your twenties or thirties or forties or fifties. Heart disease begins in the first five to ten years of life, when children get too much fat in their blood. The fat forms plaque on the inside of the arteries, narrowing them and constricting the blood flow.

I only buy products that say "no cholesterol" or "cholesterol-free."

Cholesterol (see Glossary, page 206) is only found in animal, and some seafood, products. Plants do not produce it. Because humans are animals, our bodies manufacture all the cholesterol we need to build the cell walls and produce vitamin D and bile acids. Some cholesterol, HDL (see Glossary, page 206) is actually good for us and may help prevent atherosclerosis or arterial plaque.

All fats raise your blood cholesterol levels. It doesn't matter whether the fat is saturated, unsaturated, monounsaturated, or polyunsaturated; so watch your intake of all fats.

Children get cholesterol only from meat, eggs, dairy products, and some seafood. Fats, however, come from both animal and vegetable sources. When that fat is processed in the body, it leads to higher levels of cholesterol – shortening life and lessening its quality. A cholesterol level of 180 is considered acceptable for children, but I believe that's much too high. I want children to stay with levels under 160. And the cholesterol level shouldn't ever be more than 170 when they're adults.

This is a good place to remind you that all children should have their cholesterol levels screened on a regular basis. If we only screen the high risk patients, we'll miss 50% of the children who will be at high risk for heart disease as adults because of unchecked cholesterol levels. The hidden danger for children is in potato chips, processed sweets, and candy, which are all full of greasy oil. If the package says, "No Cholesterol," it probably never had any to begin with. Cholesterol only comes from meat, poultry, fish, or dairy. But the oils – palm, coconut, cotton seed, and the rest – all elevate cholesterol levels. I'll admit olive oil and canola oil are better, but you still need to keep track of how much you're eating. Olive oil has the reputation of lowering your cholesterol. The truth is you'd have to drink a cupful each day to lower your cholesterol, and that would add 3,000 calories to your diet. You would then be in danger of death from obesity

My advice is: **"Keep fats out of your child's diet."** Stay away from meats and dairy products. Read labels. Make certain the percentage of calories that come from fat are below 15% for both you and your child.

FORMULA FOR FINDING FAT PERCENTAGE

Multiply fat grams by 9. Divide the result by the number of calories per serving.

If the label says that one serving has 150 calories with 6 grams of fat, use this formula to determine the *percentage* of fat in the product.

> 6 (grams of fat) x 9 = 54
> 54 divided by 150 (calories) = 36%

This product contains 36% fat when the recommended daily allowance should be 10 to 20%! (Sometimes, I round fat calories to the nearest ten to make the math easier in the supermarket aisles.)

---

17. I make sure that there isn't any candy in the house, and I only feed my children foods sweetened with honey or fruit juice. I can't understand why they seem so fidgety.

Honey and maple syrup are natural foods, but children should restrict their consumption of all sugars. I recommend that honey and maple syrup be forbidden for infants under 18 months. Although some experts disagree, researchers have found that children suffering from behavior disorders or learning disabilities can demonstrate dramatic improvements when sugar and junk foods are removed from their diets.

"Fruit juice sweetened" foods are equally bad. The so-called "fruit juice" is really only the sugar from the fruit, refined so that the flavor, many of the nutrients, and the fiber of the fruit are removed. What's left is plain old sugar water. "Fruit juice sweetened" foods are no healthier for you than the sugared variety.

While most products list their contents, it's still easy to be fooled. Have you ever looked at the label on a bottle of catsup? Remember that ingredients are listed according to the amount found in the product, with the predominate ingredient listed first. Look at that catsup label! You'll find sugar is listed in the first or second position. That supposedly harmless condiment is full of sugar. And I don't have to say anything about breakfast cereals, do I? Again, sugar is often right at the top of the list.

I recommend that you satisfy your child's sweet tooth with fruit. An apple, for instance, contains a high percentage of water. So the sugar in an apple is diluted and comes in small amounts. You'd have to eat a lot of apples to ingest the same amount of sugar that's in one candy bar. With the apple and other fruit, you get the added benefits of nutrients and fiber. With a candy bar, you get substances you don't want like oils and added ingredients.

Unfortunately, sugar is a food that's almost addictive. Simple sugars, like those found in processed foods, are digested and absorbed into the bloodstream very quickly.

This sudden influx of sugar elevates the level of insulin in the system. Insulin counteracts the sugar level, knocking it back down swiftly. Instead of slowly rising after breakfast, reaching a plateau, falling again before lunch, and then repeating the process throughout the day in a series of gentle curves, the rising and falling sugar levels become a jagged line of swift ascents and descents. The ingestion of simple sugars, like fruit, honey, or maple syrup, makes the body crave more sugar. The person who has doughnuts and coffee for breakfast is probably going to need more doughnuts and coffee within just a couple hours. If the sugar-eater is a child, you'll have a very busy little person on your hands. If you make note of what your children eat and how their behavior deteriorates after eating, it won't take you long to equate "hyperactivity" with food. Give a toddler sugar for breakfast, and you'll have a morning of "terrible twos" behavior ahead of you. A snack of sweet, milky cocoa with marshmallows and cookies will mean a fidgety child for the rest of the afternoon. And the child who eats sugar before bedtime will probably be cranky, whining, and awake two hours later.

Children become addicted to sugar because it tastes good and it makes them feel silly and out-of-control. I strongly suggest that you keep sugar out of your children's diets for a week or two and then evaluate the changes in behavior. Almost without exception, simple changes in the diet mean major changes in the child's temperament and behavior. In children who are already on healthy diets, it's very easy to trace. If they eat a piece of cake at a birthday party, they are awake half the night. Because their diets are cleaner, the sugar effect is noticeable immediately.

This opinion isn't shared by everyone in the medical community. But after 15 years in practice, I stand by it as do many other doctors and nutritionists.

I urge you to read all labels carefully. Know how much sugar your child is eating and try to cut out as much as you can. Children who avoid sugar don't miss it, and their parents don't miss the constant misbehavior of their sugar-eating offspring.

18. *My preschooler has a hard time with bowel movements. What can I do to ease his constipation?*

When a child hasn't had a bowel movement for a period of time and then has a painful bowel movement, he remembers the pain and tries hard to prevent it from happening again. He holds the next bowel movement for a couple of days which causes it to be even more painful, and the cycle repeats itself over and over.

But all those grunts and contorted facial and body expressions may be misinterpreted by parents as constipation when it is, in fact, the child trying to hold back and not have a bowel movement because of the painful memory of a previous bowel movement.

If you can get the child to eat fiber holding back will not be as easy and a pleasurable bowel movement may erase the bad memory. Once the cycle is broken, the child can get back on track.

A major contributor to this condition is the low-fiber American diet. This is the diet that's high in meat, cheese, and dairy products and low in grains, legumes, fruits, and vegetables, which are the fiber foods.

There are two types of fiber (see Glossary, page 208), water-insoluble and water-soluble. In the intestines, fiber (especially water-insoluble fiber) acts like a cleansing agent. It picks up water which increases stool bulk and allows it to move through the intestines more efficiently. It really is the broom that sweeps through the intestine, keeps it contracting well, and maintains regularity. Soluble fiber, such as that found in oat bran, is useful in lowering cholesterol.

In childhood, and over the course of a lifetime, a high fiber diet that emphasizes vegetables, fruits, legumes, and grains will provide other benefits besides preventing constipation. It will also decrease the incidence of diverticulosis (see Glossary, page 207) and colon cancer because it keeps the intestines clean.

Fecal matter is meant to move through the intestine and out of the body fairly quickly. When it doesn't because of low-fiber constipation, children feel out of sorts and they act out in school and at home. Later, it leads to the development of adolescent and adult diseases. It raises cholesterol and increases the absorption of fat.

Fiber in the diet is the remedy with the added benefit of making the children feel a little bit fuller and less likely to snack.

Fiber Rich Foods

Some of the best sources of fiber are:

oat bran	broccoli
wheat bran	Brussels sprouts
brown rice	cauliflower
dried figs	spinach
pears	lentil beans
raspberries	kidney beans
apples	almonds

---

19. *I am worried about the quality of our drinking water. Should I use tap water, mineral water, or distilled water for my infant?*

In April, 1993 and in 1994, the drinking water in Milwaukee, Wisconsin was determined to be unfit for human consumption for a two-week period. Well water in small or rural communities can become contaminated. Because it is impossible for parents to determine the day-to-day quality of the tap water in their community, I advise that formula be mixed with purified water found in most grocery stores and that all children drink either bottled water or water that has been run through a well-maintained, home filtration system.

I often have parents ask me if their children could drink too much water and flush the nutrients out of their system. Don't worry. You can't flush nutrients. If you drink water with a meal, the water is going to pass through the intestinal tract ahead of the solid food. If you're eating a healthy, high-fiber diet, you need to drink a lot of water to help move the fiber through your system. In fact, I encourage children to drink more water, especially in the winter when body secretions, such as mucous, become thicker. Drinking plenty of water is one of the best preventative measures for winter illnesses. Excessive drinking is rarely a sign of disease. If you are concerned, have your doctor do a urine test.

Part Five
A Practical Approach To Meals

A PRACTICAL APPROACH TO MEALS

It is unfair to present the problems with meat and dairy products, fast foods, and fats without presenting viable solutions. In this section, you will discover the secrets of a good breakfast, the importance of properly stocking the lunchbox for school, and how to best supervise your child's meals and snacks.

20. *My daughter is in third grade, and it's a fight to get her up in the morning. She's often so late she misses breakfast so she can catch the bus. Will it hurt her to skip this meal?*

As long as breakfast consists of fruit with a healthy cereal or multi-grain toast, it is the most important meal of the day for your child. She needs the energy that these foods give to help her concentrate and sustain good humor during the day. The most important thing is that the cereal be low in fat and have no added sugar or salt. It can be a simple hot cereal like oatmeal or a specially blended, low-fat granola from the health food store. Be aware that many commercial granolas are very high in fat. However, there are some new non-fat granolas showing up on supermarket shelves. Read the labels carefully! The toast can be spread with a little no-sugar-added fruit conserve. I recommend fruit instead of juice because of the high concentration of sugar in fruit juice. Fruit, which is about 90% water, has a fiber framework which slows down the absorption of sugar in the child's system. I do understand that, for convenience, juice is often the easiest choice. I would encourage children and adults always to dilute it by half with water.

Obviously, I would never suggest that breakfast, or any meal, include eggs, bacon, or sausage. These are greasy, high-fat foods that slow down the digestive system and pull blood

55

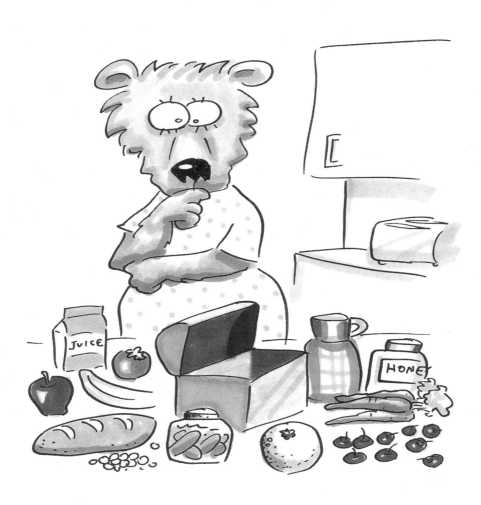

away from the brain and other organs so it can work to digest the fat. Children who eat high-fat meals can be very droopy and inattentive. When they eat lots of sugar, they have to fight the emotional instability of high and low blood sugar peaks.

In our culture, mornings are usually a hectic time with family members all rushing to work and school. This makes it difficult to sit down and have a family meal. I remember a very well-known actress whose young daughter was one of my patients. The mother came to me asking for blood tests and x-rays because her child had chronic stomach pains. When I inquired about the girl's breakfast, her mother told me she usually ate in the car on the way to school. The child was eating the proper food, but the meal was rushed and unsociable. It wasn't a time to be together as a family. When this situation was changed, the stomach aches stopped and the girl was fine.

Even if it means getting up a little earlier, plan an extra 20 minutes when your family can sit down together and get the day off to a great start at least a few days each week.

21. *I have heard that you shouldn't eat a big meal and then go to bed. Would it be better if I fed my children their biggest meal of the day at lunch?*

In many parts of the world, the largest meal is eaten at midday and followed by a siesta or nap. Most Americans don't have the luxury of sleeping for a hour or two in the middle of the day so having the largest meal of the day at noon may not make sense. Therefore, lunch should be a light and nutritious meal that includes fruit and fresh vegetables, perhaps along with a pasta or rice dish of some kind. What happens after a high-fat meal, or any large meal, is that a lot of blood flow is directed to the intestinal tract and away from the brain. This causes us to be sleepy all afternoon.

Try creating low-fat dips to go with the fresh vegetables. They make a great tasting alternative to those greasy potato chips in little bags. Liquid is also important. I don't advocate drinking milk, but a child should drink water or diluted fruit juice. With combinations of healthy foods, you can plan a high carbohydrate, moderate protein, and low-fat meal which will fuel your children throughout the rest of the day.

I'm never sure what I should pack in my child's lunchbox.

It's easier than you might think to send your child off to school with a lunchbox full of food he'll eat. Start with cold pasta in fun shapes, like corkscrews or wagon wheels. Or you might opt for a vegetable sandwich. A hummus sandwich on multi-grain bread is a winner. Then put in lots of fresh fruits and vegetables, cut into small pieces that children can eat easily. Instead of potato chips or nachos, buy nonfat whole wheat tortillas in the grocery store and cut them into wedges. Bake them in the oven and they turn into crispy little nonfat chips. Send along a container of bean dip and your child will have a healthy, tasty, nonfat snack that isn't out of place with the food his friends are eating. Again, pack water or diluted fruit juice so he gets enough liquid.

You may have noticed that I don't recommend a peanut butter sandwich, even though peanuts are relatively high in protein. There is a reason for this. Peanuts are not nuts. They are legumes, and they are very high in fat. In 1990, Consumer Reports stated that virtually all peanut butter contains aflatoxin, which is a carcinogenic mold that develops in peanuts when they are stored. Furthermore, most commercial peanut butter is full of oil, salt, and sugar. It's not much healthier than candy. A small amount of home-ground or health store peanut butter may be used from time to time, but not more than once a week.

Don't be concerned if your child doesn't eat everything, or anything, you send in his lunch box! When children are hungry, they eat. Missing a lunch here and there isn't going to hurt them. It's more important that you work with your school to ensure children in the beginning grades aren't allowed to trade foods with each other. It is self-defeating if you send healthy food and your child eats out of his friend's lunch box instead. It is the school's responsibility to monitor this and your responsibility to be a vocal parent in defense of your child's good nutrition.

Our school participates in the School Lunch Program. Is this a healthy lunch?

The School Lunch Program is a national disgrace. Motivated by lobbying forces, it's a dairy and meat oriented program which provides children with high-fat, low-fiber, high-sugar meals. Hot dogs, cheeseburgers, and french fries are common menu items. In some districts, the Program allows fast food restaurants to serve lunch in the schools, assuring that the children eat the worst possible food.

Happily, other districts are concerned about the nutritional value of the food the children are eating and they are trying to modify the program so it is healthier. These schools are setting up salad bars and offering fresh fruits, pastas, and vegetables.

The truth is that the School Lunch Program is fueled by the surplus foods of the dairy and meat industries. Our children are being fed high-fat, high-sodium meals that are sure to slow them down, clog their arteries, and set bad eating habits they'll have for life. To add to the disgrace, hot foods sit in school

SCHOOL BREAKFAST & LUNCH MENU

Monday	Tuesday	Wednesday	Thursday	Friday
	Biscuit Sausage Patty Applesauce Milk Grilled Cheese Sandwich Carrot Raisin Salad Mixed Fruit Milk	Cheese Roll Fresh Fruit Milk Breaded Chicken Coldslaw Potatoes Milk Canned Apricots	Fruited Bread Cake Milk Spaghetti w/Meat Green Salad Chilled Pears Italian Bread Milk	French Toast Fruit Cocktail Milk Sausage or Cheese Pizza Green Saland Milk Schoolboy Apple
Cold Cereal Cinnamon Toast Chilled Fruit Milk Hot Dog Vegetarian Beans Tater Tots Fruit Milk	1/2 Grilled Cheese Sandwich Canned Peaches Milk Taco Salad Shredded Lettuce Refried Beans Pan Dulce Milk Orange Wedges	Cinnamon Roll Fruit Cocktail Milk Child Care-Pancakes Rib B Que/Bun Green Salad Pineapple Tidbits Milk	English Muffin with Peanut Butter Apple Milk Chicken Nuggets French Fries Banana Oatmeal Cookie Milk	Waffle Sticks Chilled Pears Milk Sausage or Cheese Pizza Green Salad Applesauce Milk
Pancake 'N' Sauge on A Stick Mixed Fruit Milk Hamburger on Bun Shredded Lettuce French Fries Milk Chilled Peaches	Cheese Roll Fresh Fruit Milk Chicken & Rice Casserole Green Beans Fresh Apple Milk	Toast w/Peanut Butter Apple Juice Milk Ham & Cheese Sandwich Tater Tots Chilled Fruit Cookie Milk	Quesadilla Banana Milk Macaroni & Cheese Cooked Carrots Fruited Green Jello Shamrock Cookie Milk	Cowboy Coffee Bread Chilled Fruit Milk Sausage or Cheese Pizza Green Salad Mixed Fruit Milk
Biscuit Sausage Patty Applesauce Milk Corn Dog Vegetarian Beans Canned Pears Milk	Cheerios Cinnamon Toast Chilled Fruit Milk Roll Your Own Burrito Marinated Vegetable Salad Fresh Fruit Milk	Pizza Bagel Banana Milk Chicken Nuggets French Fries Chilled Pears W/W Dinner Roll Milk	Cinnamon Roll Chilled Fruit Milk Child Care-Pancakes Roast Turkey w/Gravy Mashed Potatoes Green Peas Dinner Roll Blueberry Crisp Milk	Thick French Toast w/Syrup Milk Chilled Pineapple Sausage or Cheese Pizza Green Salad Applesauce Milk
Pizza Bagel Apples Milk Hamburger on Bun Shredded Lettuce French Fries Peaches Milk	Cheese Roll Fresh Pears Milk Baked Chicken Coleslaw Dinner Roll Apple Sauce Milk	Biscuit Sausage Patty Applesauce Milk Spaghetti w/Meat Green Salad Italian Bread Diced Pears Milk	Fruit Bread Canned Pears Milk Turkey Patty w/Gravy Mashed Potatoes Green Peas & Corn Sliced Apples Roll Milk	

60

cafeterias for hours on steam tables which can destroy any vitamin content they might have had.

As parents, we must take a stand and change the program by refusing to allow our children to participate. Even the simplest lunch of an almond butter sandwich on whole wheat bread, an apple, and a glass of water is better than what is being served in the name of nutrition. It's time for parents to do some lobbying of our own!

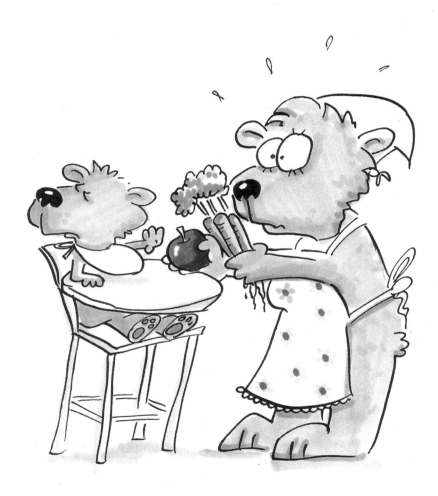

22. *My daughter frequently complains of a stomach ache at night before I put her to bed. Can it be that she's allergic to something she's eating?*

I often hear this complaint from parents. The first thing I do is take a diet history and, more often than not, I find these children are eating a lot of dairy foods and sugary desserts. This prevents the intestinal tract from working smoothly. It tries to figure out its priorities – should it digest the fat, the carbohydrate, or the protein first? The child will experience stomach cramps and hyperacidity. This increases the likelihood of sleeping problems. The blood sugar levels will bounce around, and the digestive system isn't going to work well.

Human beings are not designed like wolves, lions, or tigers. I believe that we're not meant to be carnivores. Animals who are supposed to eat meat have short, fast digestive systems. Instead, we have 25 feet of intestines in a system that works very slowly. We were designed to digest high-carbohydrate foods, not high-protein, high-fat meals. Steak and potatoes, followed by chocolate cake, is a guaranteed recipe for a stomach ache.

A family dinner is a time when everyone gets together and talks about the day. It is also an opportunity for a parent to set a good example for children. If Dad refuses to eat green vegetables, you can be certain his children won't want to eat green vegetables either. If Mom salts everything before she eats it, her children will copy her behavior. When the dining habits of the parents include meat, butter, and sugary desserts, these patterns become habits their children will follow to adulthood.

Instead, plan a balanced meal centered around a grain or pasta dish. Include a salad, vegetables, and a non-sugary fruit dessert. Serve it along with good conversation and laughter. You'll have promoted good eating habits, fed your family well, and put an end to those bedtime stomach aches.

As an inside, stomach aches can be a result of school or family stress. If good dietary adjustments don't solve the problem, probe for emotional issues.

23. I have read conflicting reports. Should I refuse to allow my little boy to eat between meals?

Research over the past decade has shown that snacking is a very healthy way to eat. In most societies, people eat six meals a day. First, they eat breakfast, and then they eat a little mid-morning snack before lunch. Between lunch and dinner they have a light snack which is called "tea" in Great Britain. Finally, they have a light, late night snack.

In America, we tend to eat just three large meals a day, each one of which seems especially designed to make us tired and physically uncomfortable.

Think of the example of animals in the zoo versus those in the wild. In the zoo, animals are fed twice a day at regular hours and are not allowed much exercise. Obesity is a constant concern. In the wild, animals graze and eat often throughout the day. They get plenty of vigorous exercise. You rarely find animals in their natural habitat with weight problems.

Like so many nutritionists, I believe we should eat six small meals a day. The term that's been coined for this kind of diet is "grazing." Like animals in the field, we should eat a little bit of the right foods whenever we're hungry. It's by far the healthiest way to keep our body's fuel level constant. Children should be allowed snacks all day long but they should be healthy snacks. Candies and pastries are out because they allow blood sugar levels to bounce up and down. These foods just slow children and make them cranky.

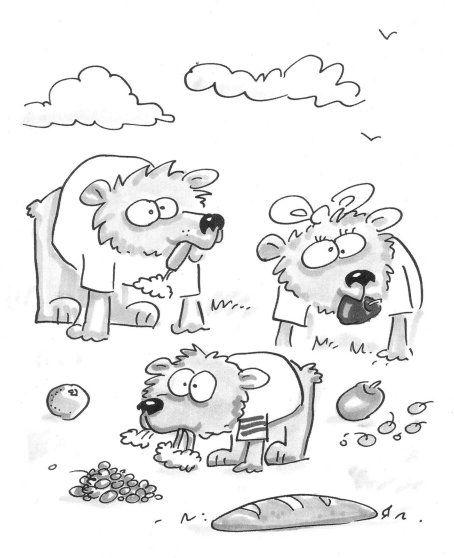

Snacks should be simple. Cut up fruits and vegetables. Make healthy dips. My daughter is often perfectly content with a small bunch of grapes or an orange. Make sure that your children know that foods are available whenever they want them. This prevents children from craving foods that aren't healthy for them. It forestalls many of the eating disorders that are becoming so common among young people in our culture. Children who eat a little of the right foods whenever they're hungry don't get fat. They don't binge. They don't fixate on food. They develop healthy habits that will stay with them throughout their lives.

The rule that I encourage for everyone is: "Eat when you are hungry and don't eat when you're not hungry." Eat as much as you feel like eating. Don't worry about set-in-stone mealtimes. With Simone, we notice that she eats a large breakfast and a small lunch and then she grazes the rest of the day. We bake potatoes and always keep some stored cold in the refrigerator so a potato can be heated up quickly when she asks for one. Meyera freezes fruit juice, or whole fruit pureé, in molds so Simone can have the pleasure of a frozen treat similar to a Popsicle® (without all the sugar found in the commercial varieties).

The over-all message is: "Be flexible, but keep the foods you have available for snacking in your home as healthy as you possibly can."

PART SIX
SPECIAL TIMES

SPECIAL TIMES

Any regimen becomes more challenging when the usual routine is interrupted by holidays, visiting in other people's homes, and traveling. In this section, you will find out how to stick to your child's healthy eating program in circumstances that are out of your day-to-day routine.

24. *My mother and I get into big arguments about the food she tries to serve my children. Do I have to stay away from her house until they're grown?*

The last thing you want to do is start fights with other family members or to keep your children away from their grandparents. We have to realize that the nutritional guidelines have changed dramatically since the time our parents were young. The old rules stressed three glasses of milk every day, meat at every meal, and desserts used as bribes for eating all those "yucky" vegetables.

In today's society, we're becoming more and more aware of how dangerous the old eating styles are. It's important that Grandma realize that the rules at your home may be quite different from what she believes is best. If she won't respect the way you're raising your children, it won't take the grandkids long to figure out they get to eat things at their grandparent's house that they're not allowed anywhere else. That's not going to be helpful to anyone.

It's time to sit down and talk to your family and tell them which foods are and are not allowed in your house. If making cookies is important to Grandma, explain the need for making them as healthy as possible. You might offer some recipes for cookies which are low in fat and sugar and high in fiber. If you

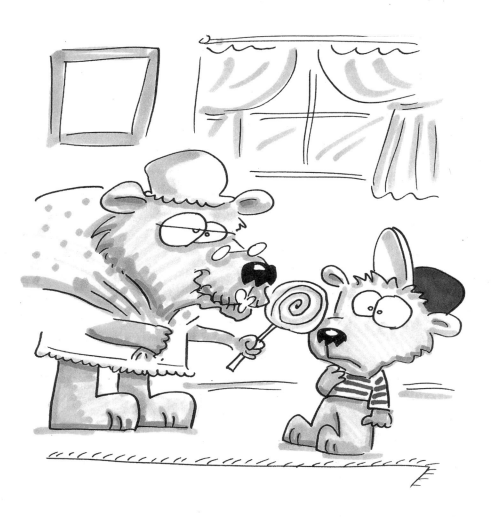

are going to be at a dinner where meat will be served and you don't want to eat it, ask if you can bring a rice or pasta casserole for your family. That way you can enjoy a meal together without compromising your nutritional beliefs. Explain that frozen yogurt is preferable to ice cream and frozen fruit desserts made without added sugar are preferable to both. You might even buy Grandma a juicer. Introduce her to fruit drinks. Stock her pantry with healthy snacks.

If it all seems too strange, you should compromise a little and meet your family half way. An occasional deviation from a healthy diet isn't going to do any permanent harm if you explain to your children that this kind of food normally is not allowed in your home. Don't ever refer to Grandma's food as "treats." You don't ever want your children to feel that sugar and fat are rewards.

What is eaten once in awhile has very little effect on your health, so don't start a family feud over this issue. Like any family disagreement, if you handle the discussion of food with humor and a willingness to negotiate, you'll have tension-free get-togethers that won't leave your children confused about who's right and who's wrong.

25. *We try to keep our junk food intake down to a minimum, but we do go to a fast food restaurant once or twice a month. It's all we can afford as a family. That can't hurt, can it?*

While there are very few times when I think you should say *never* to a child, I believe going to a fast food restaurant is one of those times. I recommend that they be avoided completely. They cook with too much oil and too much salt. While their salad bars may be attractive, they have some of the cheapest and

71

greasiest dressings you'll find anywhere. The chocolate shakes have more salt than the French fries! There is little nutritional value to what they serve. I consider them as serving heart attacks through a drive-through window.

Many fast food restaurants cook high-fat meat with high-fat cooking methods, often over a grill. The result is that fat falls on the hot flame and creates increased *free radicals* (see Glossary, page 208) in the food. These unstable oxygen molecules are charcoal-like compounds which raise blood pressure, increase heart disease, and promote the incidence of cancer.

Chicken and fish served at fast food restaurants are also often deep fried in grease. When your children want french fries, tell them how the cooks take perfectly good potatoes, soak them in yellow fat, and then deep fry them. Then they are salted before they're served. When children learn how French fries are prepared, they'll agree these potatoes don't sound very appetizing.

Many of the fast food restaurants have tried to get on the health bandwagon by putting together lighter burgers and more salad bars. Many of the greens available on these salad bars may have been sprayed with dangerous chemicals called sulfites. This substance will keep the lettuce green longer but it is highly toxic to many people. I advise all my patients to avoid sulfites.

While an occasional fast food meal won't kill you, it will begin to set patterns which will encourage the children to beg for return visits. In our family, we skip the colorful playground outside the fast food castles and we avoid the advertised toys. Instead, we take Simone to a park playground, bring our own toys, and eat foods we can be sure will never harm us.

26. *Ever since my child was born, I have begun to dread the holidays. Between celebrations and fast food, there seems to be no way to avoid eating badly. Any suggestions?*

Every parent can identify with that problem. Even if you don't pay as strict attention as I recommend to your children's diet, you've got to be concerned around Halloween about the amount and quality of candy they eat.

Holidays are times for celebrating with family and friends. It's unfortunate that we too often link some unhealthy foods with these festive periods. Just as Halloween means candy, Thanksgiving means turkey and pies. Christmas is associated with roast beef and cookies and egg nog. Even the Fourth of July has its requisite hot dogs, hamburgers, and potato salad.

During holiday mealtimes, we are careful that Simone doesn't eat anything we know will harm her and we try not to let her overdo it. However, we are definitely more lenient than during the rest of the year. On Halloween, we allow her to choose a few pieces of candy and the rest is taken to school to be counted as a math exercise. We may also eat a piece or two ourselves before they are taken to school.

A teacher at Simone's school has a unique idea. She has the children use Halloween, Christmas, Valentine's Day, and Easter candies to make clever counting games. The children paste their candy on pieces of paper to work out arithmetic problems. This way the candy can't be eaten. Instead, it's a learning tool. And the parents are very grateful for this teacher's intervention in the "candy wars."

Thanksgiving is another potentially difficult nutritional time because most people over do it with several helpings of turkey and fat-laden stuffing, along with high cholesterol pumpkin or mince meat pie. In our family, we fill up on bread, cran-

73

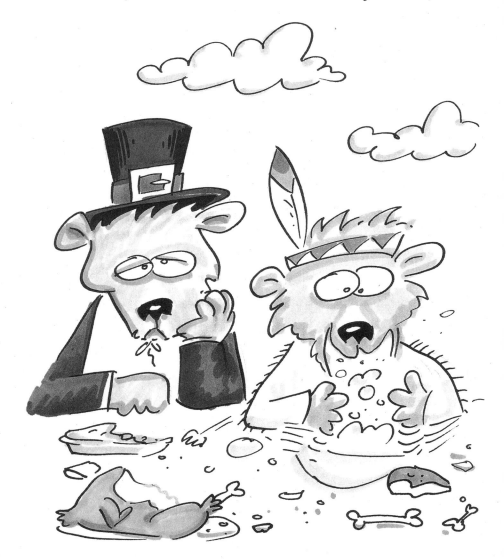

berry sauce, yams, and salad. It's easy if you're selective and you can still be part of the holiday festivities.

The Christmas holiday is a tough time to eat in a healthy way. There's a candy cane lurking around every corner and seemingly endless plates of cookies in every classroom. At our house, we focus on the joy of the season and not on the food. When we go to other homes where they may have quantities of candies, cookies, ice cream, and other unacceptable foods, we allow Simone to have one or two pieces and then say "No more."

As for the Fourth of July and Labor Day picnics, cold pasta salads, vegetable sandwiches made with whole wheat pitas, and bowls of fresh fruit all make wonderful substitutes for the more traditional American fare.

Even if I didn't have a calendar, I would know when the holidays roll around because of the increased number of phone calls I get from parents whose children are sick with abdominal complaints brought about by high-sugar and high-fat foods. There is plenty of documentation in my files to prove that children get sick more easily after they have eaten poorly. The white blood cells, which fight infection, actually move more slowly in sugary blood. This slows down the immune system so that it can't provide protection as quickly as it would in cleaner blood. If you put sugar in your gas tank, your car wouldn't run. Like an automobile, children's bodies react to bad fuel.

In our culture, we have come to expect and accept the "morning after tummy ache." It may be a common reaction to too much partying, but it's not the best way to bring up a child. I can't think of a single Holiday "goody" that's worth endangering the health of a child.

There are few things less enjoyable than a holiday vacation flight with children who've eaten a lot of junk food!

27. We're going on vacation next month, and I don't know how I'm going to keep our diets on a healthy track. Do you have any suggestions?

In the sports world, there's a phenomenon known as the "home court advantage." From the field to the locker room to the dining room, the team's home town is better set up for them than any other city. For most people, even those who pay little attention to their diet, the food at home will have less fat, salt, and preservatives than you'll find in most restaurants.

If you want the dominant memory of your vacation to be that the children were sick a good deal of the time, just allow them to eat potato chips and soft drinks in the car. Feed them from fast food restaurants, and use a candy bar to fill in the between-meal munchies.

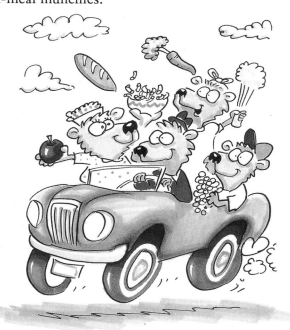

If you're travelling by car, pack healthy snacks. Fruit, cut-up vegetables, cold pasta, and slices of multi-grain bread can all be packed and put in the car. Add several small, plastic bottles of water for refreshment. If you put the bottles in the freezer overnight before you leave, the water will melt slowly and remain cool for several hours. Take a paring knife and some unbreakable containers with you, and you can stop at grocery stores along the way and replenish your supply of most things.

If we're travelling by plane, we also bring a few sandwich bags with munchies so our daughter doesn't get fretful waiting for a meal. We usually bring a quart of mineral water along in case the flight attendant isn't serving when Simone's thirsty.

Vacationing in a foreign country presents some special challenges. Whether you're going to Mexico, South America, Asia, Africa, or Europe, you're going to find bacteria and viruses that the locals can tolerate but you and your family can't. Especially when you leave the major cities, you must be very careful about what you eat and drink in order to avoid getting very sick. Fruit and vegetables need, at least, to be washed and, probably better, also peeled. Some countries require inoculations before you are allowed to visit. I have had people tell me they've travelled with supplies of antibiotics and over-the-counter stomach remedies. These medicines don't do much good.

The important thing to watch if your children do get sick is their water intake. A young child who is vomiting or has diarrhea can become dangerously dehydrated very quickly. If the symptoms don't go away within a day or if the child runs a fever, consult a doctor immediately, even if you must use sign language to be understood.

With a little care and preplanning, your vacation will be as much fun as you had hoped.

Part Seven
The Top 10 Feeding Questions Parents Ask

THE TOP 10 FEEDING QUESTIONS PARENTS ASK

There are some questions a pediatrician hears over and over again. In this section, we will put to rest your concerns about your child's eating patterns, growth and weight variances, and the effects of peer pressure on both you and your children. You'll realize that parents share similar concerns about raising healthy children, and you'll find many of those concerns answered in this section.

28. *My son isn't eating on a regular schedule. Should I be worried that he won't grow properly?*

When your baby was born, he came equipped with a well-programmed computer in his head. It provides a constant read-out of the child's condition: "January 15. 12 pounds, 15 ounces. Looking good." Furthermore, this computer has a very sensitive alarm mechanism: "11:30. All's well. Oops! RED ALERT: Hungry!" And when that alarm goes off, your baby will let you know it in no uncertain terms. You'll have no trouble understanding the message: "I NEED FOOD NOW!" Try to under-feed your baby, and he'll yell loud enough to awaken the neighbors. Overfeed him, and he'll spit up. It's a very straight-forward and very effective system.

What I'm saying is that babies know when and how much they should be eating. There is a part of the brain called the *appestat*. Just as a thermostat regulates the temperature in your house, the appestat regulates the appetite control. If your child knows that food is always available, he learns there is no reason to eat too much because he can always have more later.

But if he asks you for an apple at 4:30 in the afternoon and you say, "No, you'll spoil your dinner," then you've given the message that food is only available at certain times instead of when he's hungry. What you're setting up is a mind-set that prepares for possible problems ahead because the hunger pang isn't satisfied. Instead, if you allow your child to eat healthy foods on a demand schedule for the first three years of his life, you will have a slender, sturdy toddler who shouldn't have any eating problems later in life.

Most of the time, when I hear complaints about not eating, the children are about one year of age. Up to that point, your baby has doubled, or even tripled, its birth weight. For the next three years, the growth is going to slow down considerably. A 20-pound, 12-month-old will usually become a 38-pound, four-year-old. Obviously, his caloric needs will have decreased rather dramatically by his first birthday. As your child learns to walk and becomes more active, he uses calories more efficiently. If you offer a good, varied, and balanced diet, a child will choose to eat as much as he needs and then stop.

One reason adults become obese is that they were taught to eat more than they wanted at set intervals in the day, whether or not they were hungry. Children come into this world knowing that they should eat enough to stop the hunger pangs and no more. Instead of trying to change their behavior, we should take a lesson from it!

29. *My daughter hardly eats anything at all. I don't know how she can exist on so little food. How can I make her eat?*

We tend to forget our children are young animals. Instinct will ensure they eat enough of the correct foods. This isn't just my opinion. Classic studies have shown this to be true.

The most recent experiment was reported in 1992 in the *New England Journal of Medicine*. In this instance, researchers videotaped preschoolers who were given their choice of several different types of foods. The scientists allowed the children to eat whatever they wanted over a period of several weeks. Meticulous notes documented everything the children ate. The study showed that over a period of several weeks, each child ate a perfectly balanced diet. Instinctively, children eat enough vitamins, minerals, protein, carbohydrates, and so forth. Now, they might do this by eating nothing but rice crackers for a week before switching to another food. Or they might avoid green vegetables for six weeks, but there was nothing to worry about. Sooner or later, they chose all the elements they needed to be healthy.

I encourage parents to allow their children to eat at their own pace. If your two-year-old "eats like a bird," let her. Today she may peck like a sparrow but in a few days she may be eating everything in sight. She's just fine. A sick child is pale and listless. If your child is active and happy, how much she eats is of no concern. Just let her eat whatever healthy food she wants whenever she wants it.

30. *If I keep the four basic food groups in mind when I'm fixing meals, I won't have to worry about my children's nutritional needs being met. Right?*

I wish it were that simple. The truth is that the four basic food groups we all grew up with – dairy, meat, vegetables and fruit – are not the best foods for us. Actually, they were the brain child of special interest groups, including the dairy and beef farmers. These businessmen wanted to ensure a market for their products! Today our food group list should look quite different. Let's see why.

To begin with, in my opinion, the dairy group could better be called the *junk food group*. Studies have proven that humans don't benefit as much as was once thought from eating dairy products. Dr. Benjamin Spock, for 50 years the most beloved pediatrician in America, has stated that infants should not be fed cow's milk. The American Academy of Pediatrics announced that during the first year of life, children should have human milk for as many months as possible. And the Director of Pediatrics at Johns Hopkins University School of Medicine in Baltimore, Maryland, Dr. Frank Oski, has asserted over and over again that cow's milk is for cows and not for people.

Granted, milk and cheese do provide calcium and protein, but these benefits are far-outweighed by the dangers of eating a high-fat, high-chemical, allergenic diet. In 1992, researchers at Boston University Medical School reported that dairies were adding excess amounts of vitamin D to their milk, causing customers to become ill. In follow-up studies of dairies in five states on the east coast, 10% of the milk was found to have too much vitamin D and 61% had too little. Vitamin D regulates the body's absorption of calcium. If too little is added, you won't retain calcium. Too much Vitamin D can cause calcium to accumulate in the blood and may lead to kidney failure.

Synthetic growth hormones are now showing up in milk from some dairies'. The dangers of consuming this powerful hormone are unknown.

Researchers also found that there may be health risks from animal diseases that can be transmitted to humans through consumption of dairy products. Other studies in Canada and France have indicated that diabetes may be traced back to an immune reaction to the protein's in cow's milk. And then there are all the veterinary medicines and feed lot pesticides that are routinely found in cow's milk. I see no reason to subject any child to these dangers.

If you're worried about calcium, don't be. Have you ever seen a cow drink a glass of milk? Of course not. They get calcium from the grains they eat, and so can you. One and a half ounces of tofu will provide the same amount of calcium as a glass of skim milk. Look for calcium on the label. Some labels list it; some do not. Ounce for ounce, there is as much calcium in fresh-cooked broccoli as there is in milk.

Meat is another food group that you could eliminate from your child's diet. The protein provided by meats, fish, and poultry doesn't begin to offset the disastrous effects of fat and pollutants.

The new food groups that are being recommended for the nineties and into the new century are: Fruits, Vegetables, Grains, and Legumes (dried peas and beans). From the fruits and vegetables, you get vitamins, minerals, nutrients, and fiber. From the grains and legumes, you get protein and more fiber. Feed your children from these food groups and you'll be teaching them to eat from the very best food sources available to us. They will be lean, muscular, and energetic because they won't be filling up on fats. They will have the natural energy that comes from carbohydrates and fruit sugars instead of the frantic hyperactivity that can be triggered by processed sugar.

As a doctor, I can tell you that we're a nation of people who have a very high incidence of obesity and chronic illness. Our children would rather sit and play video games than run around outdoors. They consider fast food a treat and a gourmet dining experience. Some parents even "reward" their children with a trip to the local fast food restaurant.

We have enough new nutritional books, and medical journals to fill a warehouse, yet we continue to feed our children based on the small thimbleful of myths and misinformation that was out of date decades ago.

I encourage you to break free from the old misconceptions. Tear up the old food groups poster. It's just paid advertising for special interest groups. In its place, put up the new food groups. You'll be giving your family a gift for a lifetime.

31. *My daughter is the heaviest child in her class. She's only in second grade. Can I put her on a diet?*

Don't "put her on a diet." **Change** her diet. You'll notice the difference very quickly.

Tragically, the children of America are getting fatter. Studies reported in *Prevention* magazine found that children weighed an average of 11.4 pounds more in 1988 than they did in 1975, even though average height measurements had not changed. In other words, our children aren't growing taller. They're growing wider.

If something isn't done, these obese children will first become obese teenagers and then obese adults. Most overweight children are unhappy underachievers who learn early that you can bandage a hurt by slapping food on it. Some children will continue to eat everything in sight. Others may stop eating altogether in an attempt to get thin, developing severe eating disorders which can be life-threatening.

If you have school-age children, you shouldn't control the **quantity** of food they eat. Instead, you need to pay special attention to its **quality**. Despite your best efforts, children will trade lunches and use their allowances to buy sweet, processed foods from vending machines. It's up to you to make certain that the food that's served and stocked at your home is healthy and nourishing. It may take some time to retrain your child's taste buds so she'll reach for a slice of cantaloupe as readily as

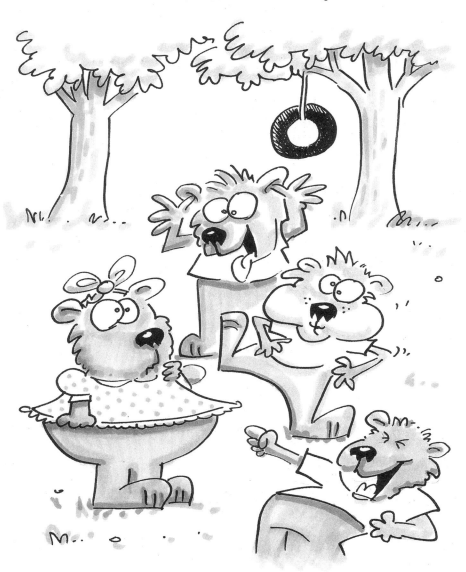

for a piece of candy, but it can be done with patience and good humor. It will be a big help if you make certain that you've swept out all the foods that are bad to eat and keep the cupboards and refrigerator filled only with the fruits, vegetables, legumes, and grains that will encourage good nutrition.

If you had started your daughter on this food plan from infancy, your feeding task would have been easier. From breast milk, a child can go to steamed vegetables and mashed fruit. Parents shouldn't use butter or cheese sauce to make these vegetables more appealing. If your child says "yuck," wait a few weeks and then offer them the food again. You'll find they may like it better as their taste buds mature. By the time a child is two or three, it will then be easy to explain that the cookies at Grandma's house aren't the kind of food you eat at your house. You aren't depriving your child of anything. This is the time to scrub out the food fallacies you were raised to believe.

It is a little more difficult if you are changing the diet of a child who has been eating junk food for six or seven years. Pediatricians have found that very few overweight children really have glandular problems. Usually the reason they are obese is that they are eating more calories than they burn off. Not only are they eating too much, they are eating fat calories that pack the pounds on quicker.

The secret I want to teach every parent is how to approach the subject of losing weight. Simply making sure that your child exercises a few times a week and eliminating a few hundred empty calories a week will result in a slimmer child. Did you know that 50% of a child's calories comes from the snacks in between meals? If you substitute fruit for candy, or carrot sticks for potato chips, you are on your way to seeing a healthier and happier child.

The worst thing you can do is talk about **diets** or **fat.** You want to keep up the child's self-esteem and prevent eating disorders. Instead of negatives, talk about food that will "make you run faster" or "help you play soccer better" or "have more fun at the beach." Make the new foods into a game. Seek out the bad ingredients in various products around the house, and throw those products away together. Teach your daughter that eating correctly is something she can take pride in. Be light hearted instead of heavy handed. Show your love and have fun!

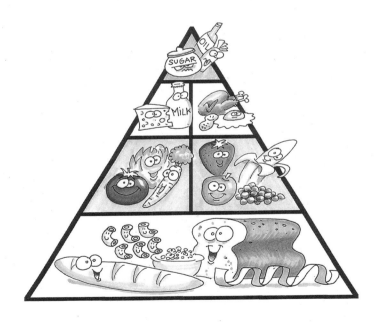

32. My son is the thinnest boy in his play group. His grandmother is always warning me that he's not healthy. How can I "put some meat on his bones?"

Grandparents always worry about children being too thin. And parents often worry about it too. Children are seldom concerned at all. The truth is that it's rare for people in this country to be too thin. Overall, the thinner people are the healthier they are and the longer they live.

If children are allowed to eat a low-fat diet of fruits, vegetables, and grains, they will end up looking thinner than the average American child. They will also be healthier than the average child.

What you want to watch closely is your child's muscle development. If he is getting adequate protein and calories, he will be growing strong muscles. If you stand back five or ten feet and take a good look at a thin child, you'll realize he looks just like a miniaturized basketball player. He's got the same body as a jogger who runs ten miles a day to stay in shape.

When judging how thin your child is, consider your family's gene pool. Generally, lean parents will have lean children and obese parents will have obese children. Usually, overweight parents and children are the result of eating the wrong foods three times a day at meals. If you are not making healthy food choices, your children will reflect the extra weight you are carrying.

Children are natural athletes. Left to their own devices, they will play hard, get enough rest, and eat the right foods in the right amounts. If well-meaning adults will just stay out of their way, they'll look like athletes throughout their childhood.

Everyone in my husband's family is overweight. Could our child have a genetic predisposition to obesity?

Yes, it's possible for genetic factors to play a part in weight gain. In my experience, however, the greatest family influence has to do with 18 years of sitting at the breakfast and dinner tables with parents who have poor nutrition habits!

33. *We have two children, and they are both very short for their age. What can I feed them to make them grow taller?*

When talking about a child's height, you have to keep in mind that pesky gene pool. At least once a week, I have a parent in my office who wants me to do sophisticated testing because their child is shorter than his playmates. When I ask the five-foot-one mother about the rest of the family, I find out that the father is five-foot-five and both sets of grandparents are under five-foot-three. With that kind of genetic background, the chances of giving birth to a future Kareem Abdul-Jabbar are pretty slim.

Just like adults, children exhibit different growth patterns. In our culture, it's not that unusual to find men six-foot-six or five-foot-five. At either height they're considered healthy and normal. We can accept the same variation in children.

The rule of thumb is that after the first year of life, youngsters grow about two inches a year throughout childhood. Between ages three and six, they grow an average of two to three inches a year. If your child is following these guidelines, very few pediatricians will recommend blood tests.

If your child has short parents, he will probably be a short adult. If your child has tall parents, he will probably be a tall adult. And if he has one tall and one short parent, he will probably fall somewhere in the middle. The formula we use to estimate the height of a full grown child is to take the parents' height in inches and apply the Rule of Five. For easy explanation, let's look at a situation where a child has a five-foot-three mother (63 inches) and a six foot father (72 inches). Here's how the formula works.

Assuming the child is a son, we'll take the father's height (72 inches) and add the mother's height **plus** five inches (68 inches). Then we add them together (140 inches), and divide by two (70 inches.) The boy will be about five-foot-ten as an adult male.

The average female is shorter than the male. So for a daughter, take the father's height (72 inches) **minus** five inches (67 inches). Add the mother's height (63 inches). The result is 130 inches, divided by two (65 inches). The girl will probably be five-foot-five when she's fully grown.

Unless there's a serious pituitary imbalance or other rare condition causing highly abnormal growth spurts or delays, there's nothing to do but watch your children grow at their own pace. Let me reassure you that height or lack of it isn't that important if the child is happy and brimming with good health.

34. *My mother bribes my daughter to eat, promising her ice cream and cookies if she cleans her plate. Now, mealtime has become a battleground. How do I get her to eat without the bribes.*

Children are very quick to pick up on the ground rules in a family. If their father refuses to eat carrots, you can believe

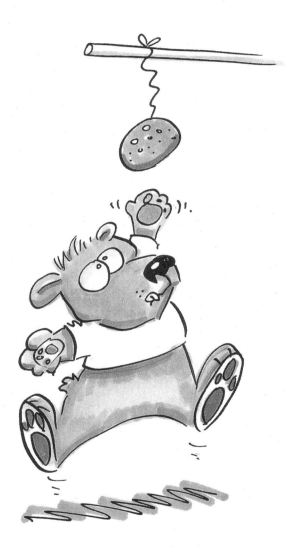

that the children are also going to turn their noses in the air when they're served. Look how frightened the broccoli growers became when the President of the United States said he refused to eat their product! If Grandma promises dessert when the food is eaten, why eat if there is no reward?

"Eat! There are starving children who would love to have that food." How many of us heard that when we were growing up? It was our first taste of guilt. Eating became a moral issue. Years ago, there was a comedian who had a weight problem. He used to say that his mother told him to eat everything on his plate because "children were starving in Europe." "So, I ate everything. And when I grew up, children were still starving, and I was fat!"

Others of us were raised with families who *lived to eat,* for whom not having enough food on the table was a mark of shame. And as adults, many of us have eating disorders and poor dietary habits, and are obese. It's time to break the pattern, and the sooner you break it the better.

With our daughter, we've been very careful to teach that food is something we need to eat if we are going to grow and have energy to play and work. Meals are sociable times when she is with at least one parent who sets the example by eating good food in moderate amounts. If Simone doesn't feel like eating, she is not pressured. If she wants to eat more than usual on a particular day, she is not reprimanded or overly praised. Food is never used as a method of reward or punishment. Eating and all that goes with it, grocery shopping, cooking, and clean-up, are treated as happy times instead of unpleasant chores.

"Eat your meat so you'll get enough protein to grow big and strong." That was the common thinking back in the 1940s, '50s and '60s when we were convinced that consuming meat and

dairy products was the only way to get protein and calcium. In the 1990's, we now know that eating such high fat foods can lead to heart attacks. We saw children with the beginnings of heart disease at one and two years of age. Nineteen-year-olds were having strokes. Men were dying in their forties from heart attacks. And it's all traceable to the food we put in our children's mouths.

I urge you to take a stand. Refuse to let your child be bribed into being overweight and risking heart disease. You may need to have a talk with Grandma, but you'll be giving your child a better treat than a piece of cake after dinner. You'll be giving her the healthy attitudes about food that will carry her through a long and active lifetime.

35. Young people have so much peer pressure to deal with that I hate to make my children feel like they're different or weird. How can I stop their playmates from teasing them because they eat strange foods?

No one wants their children to be the object of nasty teasing, however parents often react more strongly to the threat of teasing than young people do. It's your attitude about diet that will affect your children the most. If you make them proud of the way they eat and what the food does for their bodies, they will have the strength to overcome any peer pressure. In fact, my second-grader has the opposite problem. She's liable to feel sorry for people who eat meat, dairy and sugar products!

Meyera and I consciously set about to make our daughter feel that she is special because of the way she knows how to choose her foods. We used role models. Since we live in Los Angeles, she knows some very famous people who happen to be vegetarians. There are many movie stars, rock musicians, and sports figures who eat a meat-free diet. If your child is too

young to relate to these real role models, you can use Mickey
Mouse and Bugs Bunny as examples of exciting vegetarians.
Bert on Sesame Street is a vegetarian too! (We're not so sure
about Ernie, though!)

With very young children, you are in charge of what they
eat and they don't need a great deal of encouragement. By the
time they're four or five, you'll be able to do some explaining.
I tell my young patients that building their bodies is like building a house they are going to live in their entire life. You don't
want to build it out of junky materials that are going to fall
apart. Instead, you should choose strong bricks and mortar.
Slightly older children, those who are involved in sports, need
to be told that they can run faster, play longer, and grow
stronger muscles when they follow this food plan. They won't
have any problem "building themselves" up when they eat the
best food available.

One word of caution. I don't make the rules so hard and
fast that a child can't have an occasional piece of birthday cake
or Halloween candy. If the rules are too strict and unrealistic,
you're inviting rebellion. Special occasions call for special
rules. I've found that very often when children know they have
permission to do something "forbidden," they have less interest
in doing it. If your child knows he can have ice cream at the
party without having you throw a fit, he may very well turn
down the treat because there's no secondary "pay-off" in eating it.

There are some foods that we feel so strongly about that
we do say: *"We never eat this!"* Hot dogs fall into this category. I
feel there's nothing wrong with telling a child that hot dogs are
filled with pig lips and cow ears. Your child won't have any
trouble refusing to eat them and will be very vocal in telling his
friends about how disgusting they are.

If you have a daughter, by the time she is in her preteens,

the advantages of a low-fat, vegetarian diet will be very easy to explain. She will likely be the one in her class who doesn't have to worry about being overweight or fighting blotchy skin and greasy hair. She will look vibrant and healthy when many of her classmates are going through the terrors of being a teenager.

Overall, I urge you to practice moderation. Go with the flow. Let your children experiment a little at special occasions. One scoop of greasy dip on a carrot or a single piece of fudge isn't going to ruin them for life. In fact, allowing them to taste the forbidden foods will often work in your favor. To the palate that's unaccustomed to fat, these foods don't taste all that wonderful. Most children will be more than happy to go back to fruit, vegetables, and grains.

36. *My husband and I have no trouble with a vegetarian diet in our home but our parents think we're crazy and say so! How do we keep everyone happy?*

So long as there are families, there are going to be some disagreements over how the separate generations are leading their individual lives. In a perfect world, aunts, uncles, grandparents, and siblings would at least respect, if not applaud, the way we choose to raise our children. But I am well aware the world still has a way to go before nutritional awareness reaches that level. So the question becomes, how should you deal with the disapproval?

I have parents tell me that they dread holidays because the grandparents try and slip meat and sweets to the children. Grandma is insulted if everyone doesn't eat her turkey or ham. She considers it a comment on her cooking. After all, she raised you and you turned out okay, didn't you? The argument is like tic-tac-toe against a computer. You can't win.

What you can do is stand your ground. Before the event, call and discuss the situation with your parents. Gently tell them that you have very definite beliefs about what your children should be eating and you need to have your decisions honored. Explain that there are new scientific findings about the best way to eat. We now know a great deal more than we did when we were children. Just like they wanted us to grow up as healthy as possible, we want the same thing for our children. There may be some looks and muttered comments, but usually the family will rise to the occasion.

You should be aware of the mixed messages your children will be getting at these family gatherings. They are very conscious of the undercurrents, and if you don't do a little preparation, they will be confused. Tell them something like this: "Other family members don't feel the way you do about foods. They will be eating things that we know are bad for us. That's their choice, and we shouldn't say anything about it. But we know what we want to use to build our bodies. So no matter what other people say, we will choose those foods we've found are best for us."

What you don't want to do is make your family the bad guys. Tell your children: "Your grandparents are great! They just haven't learned what we have about food."

PART EIGHT
HEALTH CONCERNS

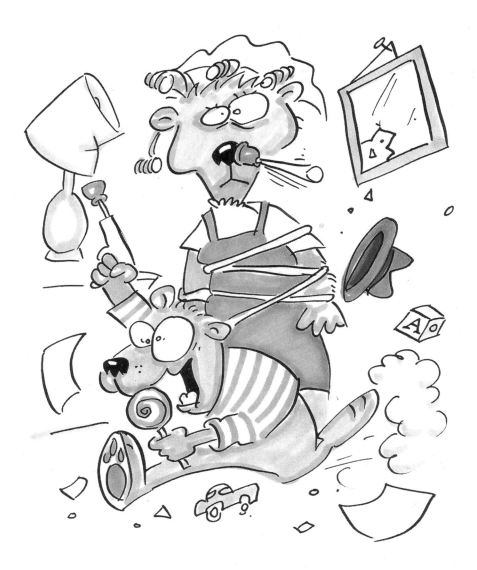

HEALTH CONCERNS

Some children do have specific health concerns that need to be addressed. In this section, we will talk about hyperactivity, anemia, eating disorders, diabetes, and dental health. You will also gain an insight into what may really be going on when you child says, "I don't feel good."

37. My son has been diagnosed as hyperactive. Can food play a part in his behavior?

Absolutely! Diet and behavior are related and there's no way to deny it.

The medical condition you are referring to is most often called Attention Deficit Hyperactivity Disorder. It probably has to do with a minor chemical imbalance in the brain which leads to hyperactive behavior. This means the child doesn't sit still well, doesn't learn well, doesn't focus well, and doesn't make friends well.

While it's still being debated, research published in respect-ed pediatric journals has established that sugar increases hyper-active behavior causing children to be jumpy and cranky. The additives in processed foods are also culprits when children have behavior disorders. My best advice is to keep your youngster on a diet of lots of fruits, vegetables, and grains. They'll feel lighter and feel more like running and playing. They're just going to be happier, healthier children all around.

103

38. *My 9-month-old daughter is allergic to both milk and dust. No one else in the family has allergies. What causes them?*

When your daughter was five-months-old, were you surprised that she couldn't walk? Of course not! Her legs weren't coordinated yet. We shouldn't be surprised if the immune system is also uncoordinated in young children.

If your infant has allergic tendencies, you want to keep her away from "foreign" proteins in her diet for the first 12 months. This means staying away from milk, eggs, and meat. When your pediatrician advises solid foods, start with fruits and vegetables. When the baby is at least seven-months-old, you can start slowly adding cereals to the diet.

As the child gets older, my advice is to keep her on this same diet, adding a greater variety of fruits, vegetables (including beans), and grain products. Children exposed to high-protein foods, especially during the first year of life, have a greater susceptibility to allergies.

If your child is a toddler and you suspect there are allergy problems with foods such as chicken, dairy, wheat, eggs, or specific fruits or vegetables, you can determine the culprit by removing the suspect food from her diet. For a few days, feed the child only a limited number of fruits and veggies. Then, add in the suspect foods one at a time. This can be as accurate as the allergist's scratch test. If you give a child some milk and she gets a stomach ache and diarrhea, then stay away from milk.

Milk allergy is the most common allergy I see in my office. Most people aren't allergic to the lactose in milk. They're allergic to the protein. That means it doesn't matter if the milk is non-fat or "lactose-reduced" or that you only give your child a couple teaspoons on her cereal. It can take only a spoonful of milk to trigger an allergic reaction which may include a runny nose, ear infection, intestinal upset, or a rash. I recommend that your family not drink milk. I consider it to be the number one allergen in our diet.

In Question 46, I discuss breast feeding and immunity, but I would like to emphasize here that we never see allergies to breast milk. The reason for this is breast milk is custom-made for the human baby. It fights infection and, if the mother is willing to pay careful attention to her diet while nursing, there should be little or no problem with digestion or gas. Breast milk doesn't "awaken" the immune system prematurely. If a child is allergic to cow's milk, the mother will have to avoid eating dairy products because their amino acid patterns will get into the breast milk and cause a reaction.

Another culprit is eggs. I see a lot of children who are very sensitive to eggs. Like milk, it's the protein that causes the problems. I believe that eggs aren't a good food for anyone because of all the cholesterol, fat, and contaminants.

Since allergies play into one another, the more you can control the better. If your child has an allergy to milk, wheat, dust, and pollen, you may not be able to protect her from dust and pollen. However, you can make her much healthier by eliminating wheat and milk. The good news is that when children eat whole foods emphasizing fruits, vegetables, and grains, you get many fewer allergies, even in families with a history of sensitivity.

39. *We've been told our son is anemic. We feed him a balanced diet with lots of meat and dairy. What causes anemia?*

Anemia is a low red blood cell count, often caused by an iron deficiency or because of bleeding. When anemia occurs early in life, it's been associated with a lowered I.Q. or learning disabilities later in life. All of these problems can be eliminated by a good diet during the first years of life.

One of the major causes of anemia in children is milk in the diet which causes micro-hemorrhaging. Small amounts of bleeding in the lower intestine increase the need for iron. If iron supplements are taken, the stomach can become irritated possibly causing more bleeding and the need for still more iron. It becomes a vicious circle.

There is no need to eat red meat to keep your children's iron intake at the proper level. Excellent sources of iron are blackstrap molasses and dark green vegetables, like spinach, kale, and broccoli.

If you follow the low-fat, no-dairy, and meat-free diet I've talked about throughout this book, your child won't have a problem with iron because he won't be losing blood after eating dairy products.

When I worked in the Emergency Room at Children's Hospital of Los Angeles, I would see chubby, pale children whose parents told me they were drinking two quarts of milk a day. The kids were getting lots of fat, and they weren't getting enough iron to replace what they were losing in their intestines. As a result, the children were fat, sallow, and anemic. We would sit down with the parents and explain that their children were drinking far too much milk. Invariably they were very surprised because they'd bought into the myth that milk was essential for proper growth. Instead of helping, they were doing their children serious harm.

Blackstrap molasses is a great sweetener that can be added to fresh baked goods or other foods. A variety of dark green, leafy vegetables can be added to salads, mixed with tofu and seasonings as a dip for lightly steamed broccoli, or used as an ingredient in soups and stews. With just a little attention to their diets, it won't be hard to keep your children from developing anemia.

The Need For Iron

The *New England Journal of Medicine* reported on a long-term study of iron deficient infants. Completed in 1991, the study showed that when infants were found to have subnormal iron levels, they had lower I.Q. scores and impaired mental functions when tested at age five.

The symptoms of iron deficiency include listlessness, irritability, headaches, and, in some cases, a craving called "pica" which causes the child to eat dirt, paint chips, and other non-food substances.

The absorption of iron is maximized by consumption of vitamin C at the same meal as iron-containing food.

---

40. *It seems as if one of the children is always sick, –nothing really serious, just the normal childhood stuff. Is there any way to avoid this?*

The most common complaints I treat in basically healthy children relate to the upper respiratory system, the stomach, and the intestines.

Colds are going to happen to all children occasionally. If doctors knew how to cure colds, maybe we'd be able to prevent them. What we can do is advise parents to keep the children away from dairy products which will make the cold seem much worse than it is because they increase allergic response and may thicken mucous in the system. Unlike adults, youngsters don't localize infections very well. They rarely have just a stuffy nose or right ear infection. They tend to get runny noses, runny stools, runny eyes – runny everything all at once. If children are drinking a lot of milkshakes or hot cocoa made with milk, they're going to have more mucus both in the sinuses and throat and they're going to be much more uncomfortable.

One of the ailments pediatricians see most often is stomach flu. When children have a viral stomach episode, the intestines tend to slow down or stop. As a result, they don't digest foods that require effort. In this situation, you have to treat the intestines gently and heal them with a "zero protein diet." Even after the flu has run its course, continue on the zero protein regimen for another 24 hours. Offer diluted juices, a little apple sauce and mashed banana, steamed yams and carrots, and other fruits and vegetables. The child will be well-nourished and won't become dehydrated. If you offer a higher protein load, your child will vomit and have much more debilitating diarrhea.

Many people don't realize that the definition of diarrhea has to do with the frequency of stools, not their consistency. One or two loose stools a day isn't diarrhea. In fact, a balanced grain, vegetable, and fruit diet will cause stools that are soft and easy to pass. That's healthy.

When children are having eight to ten stools or more a day, they have diarrhea. It is most often caused by a virus and will be aggravated by a bad diet. The nutrients pass straight through the system. Dehydration is a concern. The answer is to allow the intestines to rest in order to avoid a severe situation which could require hospitalization and intravenous fluids.

There is a common misconception that fruits cause diarrhea. In fact, fruits and vegetables are very helpful when dealing with diarrhea. When they get into the intestine, fruits and vegetables absorb water and solidify watery stools. Like adults, children should have loose, easy-to-pass bowel movements, not hard pebbles or chunky stools. A well-nourished child will have these loose bowel movements up to three times a day.

Constipation is the opposite of diarrhea, and it's quite common in children from two to five. Because the stool is hard and uncomfortable to pass, the children hold it in longer. This aggravates the problem. Very often the cause for the chunky and painful stools is an inadequate intake of fluid or fiber. The intestines are not meant to digest high fat, high protein food because it slows them down. Stools don't move through the intestines with the cleansing action needed and actually dry out, narrowing the width of the intestinal tube. You have to flush them out, and a high fiber diet is the best way.

When children drink lots of water and diluted fruit juices (prune juice is the best) and eat plenty of oatmeal, rice, and pasta along with fruits and vegetables, constipation is almost never a problem.

41. *My son was just diagnosed as having childhood onset diabetes. There's never been any diabetes in our family. How can this happen?*

Every day there is more evidence that milk in a child's diet may increase the incidence of diabetes. About 20 percent of children carry a gene that may predispose them to diabetes. If those children are fed cow's milk, it may actually accelerate the tendency to develop the disease. While still debated by some experts, this is a sound theory based on solid scientific fact.

When a child has diabetes or pre-diabetic tendencies, we know that an optimal diet helps.

When a pregnant woman is diagnosed with borderline gestational diabetes, the first thing her doctor will do, before prescribing any medication, is to change her diet. Like heart disease and hardening of the arteries, adult onset diabetes can have its beginnings in childhood, even though it may not manifest until 50, 60, or even 70 years later. It is a disease of abuse. A good diet in childhood sets the stage for optimal pancreatic function throughout life.

42. My neighbor's child was just diagnosed with cancer. She always seemed so healthy. What causes this in children?

There is no one simple answer to why a child gets cancer. In most situations, we can only make educated guesses.

What we do know is that we can reduce the rates of cancer in children and adults. Breastfed babies have less teenage cancer. We have to keep youngsters on the proper diet, keep their colons clean, expose them to fewer additives and to fewer cancer-causing agents (carcinogens). Cooked meat has more carcinogens than cooked fruits and vegetables. A diet high in fruits and vegetables and grains keeps the colon clean and is associated with lowered incidence of breast, colon, and cervical cancers.

Pesticides have been linked to cancer in studies of laboratory animals. To reduce your child's risk of exposure to these significant known carcinogens, make every effort to raise your children on a diet of organic fruits, vegetables, and grains that were raised without chemicals either deposited in the soil or sprayed on the crops.

If we raise our children without processed, pesticide-ridden foods and teach them good eating patterns, they'll enjoy the benefits throughout a lifetime.

43. My daughter is only ten but she's already obsessing about her weight. She only eats a few bites of food a day. Should I worry about eating disorders?

Eating disorders have become a major problem in American society. We've raised our children to obsess about food. Magazines, television programs, and even newspapers blare the message that "you can't be too thin." It's fashionable to be unrealistically skinny. These same magazines and newspapers report on well-known models, actresses, and other celebrities, who have severe problems with anorexia and bulimia. A young girl then turns on the television and sees very thin people selling fattening foods. It's just not fair!

Since thin is in, fat is the obvious rebellion. Stress is resolved with food. Anger is appeased with food. Sadness is assuaged by food. Unhappiness shows up on the hips in a heartbeat, an easy feat given the typical high-fat, low-fiber diet.

When you're raising children, you must never emphasize weight. Instead, talk about strength, fun and healthy foods, and strong muscles and sturdy bones. The way to help a child stay at the correct weight is to change her diet to healthier foods and her lifestyle to one that is more active with plenty of outdoor exercise. If you have a seven-year-old who is somewhat overweight, make sure she doesn't put on any more pounds, and she'll eventually grow tall enough to fit the weight she's carrying. Growing children should never lose weight. Instead, they should get taller.

The two most common eating disorders are bulimia and anorexia nervosa. Both are more common in girls because boys are less affected by societal pressure to be thin. Also, boys tend to be more physically active than girls.

Bulimia is the act of binging (eating uncontrollably) and then immediately purging (making yourself throw up). Very quickly, the enamel on the teeth begins to be affected, and, in time, the esophagus can be damaged by repeated exposure to stomach acids. Sometimes you'll find bite marks on the knuckles because they've put their fingers down their throat to gag. Bulimics tend to spend a lot of time in the bathroom right after meals. Eventually, because they're not getting any nutrients from their food, bulimics become very thin.

If you ask a ten-year-old girl how she sees herself, usually you'll hear that she's "too fat." In our society, many ten-year-olds have already been on self-imposed diets.

When a child develops anorexia nervosa, she stops eating altogether. This means the child doesn't eat enough to maintain good muscle mass. Because it has no food to digest, the body literally begins eating itself. In a short time, anorexia sufferers become emaciated. They lose the rounded contours of the shoulders. They have no buttocks. Their legs are spindly because the thigh and calf muscles waste away. Their electrolytes (see Glossary, page 207) go out of balance, and they may stunt their growth and delay puberty. In worst case scenarios, as with singer Karen Carpenter, anorexia can be fatal.

Amazingly, anorexics firmly believe they are carrying too much weight. They will never be thin enough. It becomes impossible to swallow more than a bite or two of food at a meal.

Both these diseases result from attaching too much importance to food, making it a reward or punishment or source of comfort. You should never send a child to bed without dinner as a punishment or give an extra cookie as a reward. This is how you raise a child who grows up thinking that's what food is all about.

We don't have to celebrate with food, and we don't have to deprive ourselves. You shouldn't deliberately eat less on Tuesday because you ate too much on Monday; you should only eat to satisfy hunger. You don't have to clean your plate. You don't have to miss dessert because you didn't finish your salad. Instead, teach that food is nothing but fuel. It's not that important in and of itself. Food's only purpose is to properly fuel the body and promote good health.

44. *Could you give us some advice about diet and our children's teeth?*

The things I've been saying about diet throughout this book hold true for the issue of your children's dental health as well. The idea that we have to drink cow's milk to grow strong teeth is totally false. The diet of fruits, vegetables, legumes, and grains will give your children all the nourishment they need to grow healthy teeth. Staying away from sugar and processed foods will also help prevent tooth decay.

What about fluoride?

The issue of fluoride has been around for about 40 years now, with communities arguing about whether or not the water supply should be fluoridated. There is some thought that we could be in danger today of getting too much fluoride. Fluoride toothpastes, combined with the small amounts of fluoride that occur naturally in the drinking water, can cause a condition called fluorosis. Too much fluoride in the diet can cause youngsters to have either permanent brown spots or little lightened areas on their second set of teeth.

If a child eats fluoridated toothpaste off the toothbrush, and all children eat toothpaste up to the age of two or three, they can get 10 times more fluoride than they should in any given day. Current thought is that fluoride treatments by your child's dentist should begin at about age three. Fluoride supplements can be started between ages two to four years.

My advice is to feed your children a healthy grain, legume, vegetable, and fruit diet, teach them to take care of their teeth with frequent brushing and flossing as they get older, and make your dentist a friend who is visited regularly.

PART NINE
IMMUNITY

IMMUNITY

What better gift could you give your children than immunity from childhood disease? In this section, the secrets of immunity are revealed, beginning with the earliest days of your baby's life. Specific instructions will help you protect your child from day one to adulthood.

45. *What can I do to give my child immunity from some of the health problems of childhood?*

Even before your son or daughter is born, accept the fact that there are a certain number of illnesses and accidents that are a normal component of raising a child to adulthood. There is no way to raise a healthy, active, and psychologically stable youngster without at some time having them in danger from falls, cuts, or viruses. It goes with the territory.

What you can do is put the best fuel possible into your children and make sure that they have a body that will heal quickly no matter what unhealthy incident befalls them. If your child breaks an arm falling off the monkey bars at the school playground, you want the bones to heal well and be strong. If a bad scrape on your first grader's knee becomes infected, you want the immune system to be ready to shift into high gear and fight the bacteria. If an ear infection sends your toddler's fever soaring, you want her to have the strength to fight the disease.

If your child's blood stream is loaded with sugar, the white blood cells will be slowed down in their race to the site of the infection. The cookies and candies that are everywhere during the holidays can ruin a ski vacation by weakening the immune system. At Christmas, I get calls from all over the country from parents whose children have fallen ill on vacation. They've eaten a lot of sweets and rich foods, and their bodies are in the overload mode. The youngsters are stressed because of the new environment away from home, and they get hit with a virus. On the wrong diet, they don't have the strength to defend themselves against it.

So boost your child's immune system by bringing apples on the plane instead of candy. Offer water instead of soda. Serve pasta instead of pot roast. Have your youngsters eat better, and their immune systems will work better. They'll get sick less often and recover more quickly. You won't think these are extreme nutritional measures if you've ever been on vacation with a toddler who has stomach flu! We know this works for us adults. Let's do it for our children.

46. *I would like to nurse my baby but, as a working mother, I'm concerned about the issue of time and convenience. Is it really necessary to breastfeed or will formula be sufficient?*

Whenever possible, human infants should be fed human milk, just as cow's should be fed cow's milk and goats should be fed goat's milk. Everything about human breast milk is perfect for your baby.

If you look at the label on a can of formula, it looks as if you're reading the label on a candy bar without the chocolate wrapped around it. Formulas have either cow's milk or soy milk, mixed half and half with water, with added coconut oil, added sugar, added vitamins and preservatives and, most recently, added amino acids. Formula is the beginning of the junk food habit.

Your baby will thrive on your milk. It's a continuation of the protein, amino acid, carbohydrate, and fat patterns the baby grew on during pregnancy. If you look at human breast milk under a microscope, you can see millions of white blood cells moving around ready to fight "the infection of the day." You can actually study the antibodies the mother has left over from her own childhood and those she's developed to fight the viruses of today. Breast milk decreases the incidence of allergies in babies and probably decreases the incidence of diabetes, respiratory illnesses, and intestinal problems. Processed formulas have never and will never be a good simulation of breast milk.

But how can I breastfeed while I have a full time job?

A working mom can use breast pumps to provide a supply of mother's milk for her infant when she is away at work. Breast milk can be refrigerated and used for up to 72 hours. However, it is necessary for the mother to use the breast pump two or three times during the day at work to keep up her milk supply for her baby. Otherwise, her milk supply will fail or she can experience painful feelings of fullness. Medela, Inc., a breast pump manufacturer in McHenry, Illinois, has a pump rental and education program for companies interested in supplying breast pumps for their women employees. Or women can call Medela's toll free number, 1-800-435-8316, to find a pump rental location in their area.

What if I'm not able to produce enough milk?

If you don't think you have enough milk, then you don't have enough information. If you think you don't have time or proximity during the day, then you don't have enough information. If you are discouraged because you are having trouble breastfeeding, you don't have enough information. In many ways, breastfeeding is as important for the mother as it is for the baby. Not only does it promote a closer bonding with the baby, but mothers who breast feed for at least six months have a lower incidence of breast cancer. I wish all obstetricians and pediatricians would encourage mothers to breastfeed and put them in touch with members of the LaLeche League. Call 1-800-LA-LECHE, and you'll get a wealth of helpful and caring information.

I plan to breastfeed for at least the first six months. What should I include in my diet?

Mothers who are breastfeeding need to eat a balanced diet. The baby will take 500 to 1000 calories a day, so you should be able to eat well and still lose the weight you gained during pregnancy. The cleaner your diet, the fewer pollutants you take in with your food. A study published in the *New England Journal of Medicine* in the late 1970's showed that vegetarian mothers have the cleanest breast milk in terms of 17 different industrial pollutants. If you are eating meat and dairy products, your pregnancy is a good time to stop eating them so that your milk will be the very best you can feed your baby.

We are adopting a baby, and I will be using formula. What should I be concerned about?

You will need to consult with your pediatrician to find a formula that will be as healthy as possible for your baby. There are a fair number of infants who are sensitive to cow's milk formula and an equal number who are sensitive to soy milk formula. Recently manufacturers have come out with so-called hypo-allergenic formulas. However, I haven't found them to be what they're purported to be, and I don't recommend them.

Work closely with your doctor, and try to find a formula you can stick with throughout the first year of life. Changing formulas will only upset the baby's system while he's adjusting to them.

My very best advice is use formula only as a last resort. If you do use a soy-based formula, make certain that it is made from organically-grown soybeans.

Sometimes there is a family member or friend who can supply your baby with breast milk. If not, the La Leche League may be able to put you in contact with a mother who would be willing to donate breast milk to you for at least the first few months of your baby's life. Ask!

PART TEN
PHILOSOPHY

PHILOSOPHY

There will always be people who disagree with how you are feeding your children. In the following pages, you will learn non-threatening techniques for explaining your new way of eating.

47. *How do I talk to my children about the importance of good food in ways that they can understand?*

You have to talk to children at the level they are on intellectually. When three-year-olds and four-year-olds come in for their check-up, we talk about how they can grow bigger and stronger muscles if they eat vegetables and spaghetti and fruit. I tell them that if they eat cookies and candies and greasy foods, they won't be able to jump and play the way they'd like. At home, the parents can then build on "what the doctor told you."

A couple of years later, I talk about specific activities that the child may like such as baseball, soccer, swimming, or whatever. Then I ask, "Do you think you'll be able to run and kick better if you eat French fries and milkshakes or if you eat vegetables and fruits?" They have no trouble coming up with the right answer. We talk about which fruits and vegetables are their favorites, and I assure them that eating those vegetables is just the right thing to do if you want to be the best player on the team. I stress the fact that they're "big kids now" and they know better than to eat sweets and meat. I say, "Only little kids think that's good for you!" I also encourage them to eat backwards once in awhile. Have cereal for dinner, and spaghetti for breakfast. It's fun, and it makes the day's meals more interesting.

It's effective to put mental pictures in a child's head. I call fast food hamburgers "greaseburgers" and refer to cheese as "chunks of fat." We describe how butter looks if you leave it in the hot sun so it gets "all gushy." Ask your six-year-old if he'd want to rub that greasy butter all over his face and hair. Of course, he wouldn't. So explain that's just what he's doing when he eats a hamburger and fries, only he's rubbing it on the inside. Yuck!

As the child gets older, we talk about "brain food" and the benefit to his grades if he eats the right way.

If you have teenagers, you can talk about how they look. Kids who eat low-fat, low-sugar vegetarian meals don't have acne, sallow skin, or greasy hair. They look vibrant and alive. They are full of energy and can really enjoy school and extra-curricular activities. No one wants a date who's covered in make-up to hide bad skin and who's too tired from an unhealthy diet to enjoy several hours of dancing.

Remember, use examples with **immediate** rewards. Young people don't think in terms of tomorrow. They live and breathe for today. They're more interested in the benefits at 15 than 50.

48. *What can I do to help my sixth grade daughter raise her self-esteem?*

Self-esteem in children is an issue that is finally beginning to be recognized as an important cornerstone in healthy development. If you, as a parent, are careful to nurture self-esteem in your child from the day she's born until the day you die, you will have given her a wonderful gift. At whatever age, infancy through adulthood, humans need to believe that they are lovable, respected, and worthy. No one can implant that belief more effectively than parents.

126

When you raise your child to eat well so she has few illness-es and more than enough strength to cope with whatever her day brings, you are empowering her. She becomes very confi-dent of her ability to handle whatever may come up.

One of the worst impediments to self-esteem is obesity. When a child feels uncomfortable with her body and thinks other children are laughing at her, she feels unworthy. She becomes defeated and will often turn to junk food for solace from the very condition the junk food caused in the first place.

Teaching your child to eat correctly and exercise more gives her a sense of power. Even at ten or 11, she's in charge of her own body and she's proud of what her body looks like and what she can accomplish with it. If you can instill this feeling in a child, you have a winner – a kid no one can hold back even for an instant!

49. *I'm convinced! Now I have to convince my family. How do I change our diet most effectively?*

Did you ever hear the riddle, "How do you eat an ele-phant?" Actually, I'd prefer it to be "How do you eat a water-melon?" In either case, the answer is "One bite at a time." And that's how I'd like you to look at converting from the typi-cal American diet to one that is centered around fruits, vegeta-bles, grains, and legumes. You need to make this a family pro-ject, and that includes winning over your spouse who may prefer meat and potatoes.

Begin by serving the same foods you've always made, but cut out the oils and sugars whenever possible. If you're serving steak and French fries, make the piece of steak smaller, and for the fries, substitute a baked potato. Replace the sour cream and butter with yogurt and chives, and add a colorful vegetable to the meal. Gradually, move to rice and pasta dishes in which the meat is more of a flavoring than a major ingredient. If you take it slowly and don't shock their sensibilities, even the most dedicated meat muncher will begin to enjoy the new foods. By the time he realizes you're doing something different, he'll feel much better, and he'll think it was his idea in the first place!

You'll find there are tastes that your children don't like. Broccoli or cauliflower may not cause them to cheer when it first shows up on their plates, so try combining them with other tastes. Add the new vegetables to a familiar salad or pasta. Remember that fresh vegetables always taste better than canned or frozen. Keep them crisp and not mushy.

You can do the same sort of substitution over time with foods like chili. Gradually reduce the meat, increase the beans, and perhaps add vegetables until no one really notices the difference.

It's up to you! Just don't restock the greasy snack foods when you go to the store. Buy more from natural food and health food stores and less from the supermarket. Replace mayonnaise-laden egg salad with a flavorful tabbouli made with grain, green onions, tomatoes, vinegar, and a little olive oil. You can find the complete mix in a box at most grocery stores. Instead of French onion dip, have hummus ready as a dip for carrot sticks and zucchini slices. In place of a bowl of oily potato salad, provide cold pasta with seasoned low-fat dressing. For dessert, serve a plain baked apple, stuffed with cinnamon and raisins, instead of a fat-laden apple pie.

You **can** convert your family from the old ways to the optimum diet. It's going to take a little effort on your part but the rewards will be greater than anything else you could wish for your family. Optimum health and well being.

PART ELEVEN
MEYERA'S KITCHEN

MEYERA'S KITCHEN

This final section has been contributed by my wife, Meyera. Here you will find down-to-earth suggestions for how to prepare your kitchen and your family for good food today and always. Meyera leads you by the hand through restocking the pantry, shopping, and cooking. All you have to do is follow her 14-Day Transition Plan and you will find your conversion to a vegetarian lifestyle uncomplicated, delicious, and fun!

50. *I think I have to do a lot of retraining in the kitchen. Where do I begin?*

Let me make one thing very clear. I am a pediatrician and not a chef. Happily, I married a remarkable woman who thinks the way I do about food and who once owned a highly-acclaimed, vegetarian restaurant. She more than makes up for my deficiencies in the kitchen. Meyera will respond to the remaining questions in this book.

MEYERA:

I'm happy to answer! I've been cooking low-fat, low-sugar vegetarian meals since 1967. It was certainly a change for me from the way I learned to eat as a child. Growing up, we ate meat at least three times a week for dinner. Canned and processed foods were staples. But we always had salad and that was my favorite part of the meal.

When I decided to change my diet, I wasn't living at home any longer. I was on my own, free to experiment and learn. It wasn't as hard as I expected it to be. I learned by trial and error because at that time there wasn't a wealth of vegetarian and fat-free cookbooks in the stores. Today there are dozens of books

131

you can refer to for help. I started by using ethnic cookbooks, simply leaving out the meat.

For most Americans, vegetarianism is a diet of subtraction and addition. The cooking techniques are very much the same. You steam, sauté, stew, bake, and boil, but you subtract meat, fish, poultry, dairy products, oils, and margarine. You also cut way back on the sugar, honey, and artificial sweeteners. This leaves you with a lot of empty plates. That's where the addition comes in.

To fill those plates, you add fresh vegetables, fruits, and dishes using dried beans and grains. You also find new and varied uses for whole grain pastas. The plates are full again. Your family is satisfied. And you've made major steps in improving their health.

Many references have been made about how important it is to read labels. Can you give some advice on how to do this?

By law, food labels must state the contents of the product. Now you can easily determine the amount of calories, fat, carbohydrate, cholesterol, and sugar in most packaged foods. You can also determine the relative amounts of each ingredient by reading the listing of contents. Each ingredient is listed from the greatest to least amount. Therefore, if a label on your loaf of bread lists corn syrup as a major ingredient, you know that you're not getting a healthy product no matter how many whole grains it purports to have.

You also want to be on the lookout for names you can't pronounce. We'll always have to deal with some additives to preserve our food, but we don't want to consume any more than is absolutely necessary. Generally, the fewer ingredients on the label the better. If you can easily recognize and pronounce them, there's usually even more of a benefit.

Salt is often added to food as a preservative, so look for the word "sodium" or any derivative of it. Some foods, like soy sauce and most bouillon, are full of salt. In some stores, however, you can find bouillon without the salt. Soy sauce manufacturers, unfortunately, offer only a lowered-salt rather than a no-salt alternative. I use soy sauce in my recipes but I have marked it "optional" for those who want to avoid sodium.

Sugar in food is hidden under names like: maltose, sucrose, dextrose, fructose, and corn syrup.

Oils are also often added to foods. In an effort to reassure the public about the dangers of cholesterol, many manufacturers have replaced lard with palm, coconut, or cottonseed oil. These oils are just as dangerous as lard. You should read the labels carefully to determine that there isn't any added oil.

Monosodium glutamate and sulphur dioxide are also ingredients you want to avoid. Monosodium glutamate is the infamous MSG that Oriental restaurants once used with a heavy hand. And it isn't just used by Oriental restaurants. Accent®, a food enhancer sold in every supermarket, is pure MSG. Many people are very sensitive to this salt that comes from one of the amino acids found in proteins. The person who has trouble with this ingredient may experience nausea, headaches, heartburn, and that "stuffed" feeling that is common after a large Chinese restaurant meal. MSG is also found in some soy sauces.

Sulphur dioxide is a sulfating agent that is commonly used as a preservative. By law, all sulfating agents must now be identified clearly on the package, because some people may have severe reactions ranging from shortness of breath to shock and coma. Sulfites are commonly found in wines, beer, dried fruits, and in many salad bars; they keep lettuce and other vegetables looking crisp. Even though it is illegal, some butchers use sulfites to keep meat red and fresh-looking.

With practice, you will become proficient at reading labels and knowing which foods are good for you and your family. You can make a game for your children out of reading the labels. Not only will they become proficient at finding the unpronounceable synthetic ingredients, they'll also learn to look for the order in which ingredients appear. It won't be long before your children will know that if "Sugar" is listed first, this is a product your family doesn't want to eat because sugar is the main ingredient.

You'll find that as your skill and confidence in preparing vegetarian meals increases, you'll be using fewer processed foods and making more meals with fresh, organic foods that have no pesticides or additives contaminating them.

On the following pages, I will share with you some of the Gordon family favorite recipes. You'll find these foods easy to prepare, delicious to eat, and nutritious for children and adults. I've also provided a guide for restocking your pantry, ideas for packing school lunches, cooking tips, and a 14-Day Transition Plan to lead you to a healthier diet. Enjoy!

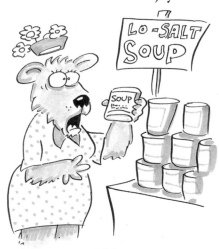

PANTRY RESTOCKING GUIDE

1.   Go through your pantry and refrigerator and get rid of everything that doesn't work with your new lifestyle. I would encourage you to donate all of the foods you are cutting our of your family's diet:

> Cereals with sugar
> Processed foods
> Canned foods with additives
> Anything containing animal oils
> Pastas with eggs
> Cheeses

2.   Now go to the health food store near you. If there isn't a health food store that's convenient, go to your neighborhood supermarket. You'll find most of the foods you need.

3.   Live by this **Golden Rule of Nutrition:**

Read EVERY label!

This rule applies even in health food stores! Become accustomed to knowing the ingredients in everything you eat. If you can't pronounce it, it's probably not good for you! Stay away from products that list sodium, sugars (including words that end in "ose"), and all meat, poultry, and fish extracts.

4.   Start by stocking up on the basics:

> Short grain brown rice
> Polenta (corn meal)

Lentils
Split peas
Kidney beans
White beans
Garbanzo beans
Cans of organic chopped tomatoes
Tomato paste – no salt
Pastas – varied (without eggs) (Wagon wheels,
      shells, rotini; wholewheat, if possible)
Udon noodles (Japanese – great with a stir-fry)
Spaghetti in various sizes
      Quinoa pasta (high in calcium)
      Amaranth pasta (high in iron)
      Oatmeal
Granola (no-fat)
Baked goods/breads – oil and salt-free
Fruits/vegetables (Buy the very best so your
      kids can get used to the fresh taste.
      Whenever possible, buy organic produce.
      It's much healthier.)

5.   Recycle! Buy recycled paper products. Reuse plastic bags.*
Bring canvas sacks with you. Teach your children to recycle,
and ask them to help. Become a compulsive environmentalist.

Good Luck!

* *Except for bread bags which contain printing ink which may conta-minate your foods.*

GENERAL TIPS

√   Make more than you'll need for a particular meal or snack. Leftovers can taste great!

√   Prepare soups, sauces, cooked beans, etc. in large amounts and freeze them. Make sure you carefully label and date the packages when you put them in the freezer. I use a grease pencil that you can buy at any stationery store which washes or rubs off easily so you can reuse the container.

√   Keep a supply of pastas and grains on hand. They're so easy to use as a base for an interesting meal. Sometimes, Simone snacks on plain cooked pasta or I pack leftover pastas in her lunchbox.

√   You may notice a repetition of ingredients in the following recipes. I use a lot of the same vegetables as a base for a meal. While the ingredients are similar, the tastes are very different depending on how the food is cooked and seasoned.

√   Alter the ingredients you add as well as the seasonings. You can change the beans or rice in a vegetable soup, and it changes the whole dish. Add basil and oregano and tomato, and it will be quite different from the soup you made with the same base and seasoned with parsley and thyme a week or two earlier.

√   To thicken soups without flour and milk, purée one half of the basic mixture and mix it back in with the unpuréed vegetables and broth.

137

√   We like some simple foods like a hearty vegetable stew served with a delicious bread and a salad. Good bread makes any meal more interesting. Buy partially baked breads, and serve them hot out of the oven for dinner. Watch the labels for oils!

√   Use one third of the usual amount of oil on everything. Don't fry anything. Grill or lightly sauté, preferably in non-stick pans. A little oil can go a long way.

√   Season with lemon juice and honey.

√   Instead of sugars, add fruit juices or fresh and dried fruit.

√   Instead of dairy products, use soy products or rice milk. If you must have eggs, use only the whites. A dab of yogurt can replace butter on baked potatoes.

14-DAY TRANSITION PLAN

Note: This plan is not meant to be a set-in-stone guideline. You can spend a week making the changes suggested for one day, or you can move ahead even faster. You need to be confident with the changes, and make them at your family's most comfortable speed.

In deference to working mothers and the needs of running a busy household, we've started the 14 Day Transition Plan on a Friday so that you can have a weekend to prepare the kitchen and pantry for the changes that are coming.

DAY 1 – FRIDAY

Preparatory time. Explain to your family that you're going to be more food conscious. Ask your children for suggestions or a list of their favorite healthful foods. Prepare a dinner that has little or no meat. Go through your cupboards, the pantry, and the refrigerator, and give away all foods that have preservatives, sugar, or fat. Local shelters will welcome boxes of packaged and canned foods. (This includes cheeses. You can replace them with no-fat cheeses for the time being.) If your children are old enough, make this a family project.

DINNER (1)*	Stir Fry Vegetables w/Brown Rice
	Your Favorite Salad
(2)	Baked Apples w/Strawberries

* *Numbers indicate a recipe.*

139

DAY 2 - SATURDAY

Begin to cut down on your portions of red meat, pork, and veal. Increase the size of your portions of vegetables and starches. Make a shopping list for the health food store. Go shopping with the children, and let them read the labels so they begin to understand the ingredients. Buy healthy substitutes for meat products: beans, short grain brown rice, vegetable pies, soy hot dogs, etc. (See Pantry Restocking Guide on page 135).

BREAKFAST		Glass of Fresh Orange Juice or Orange Juice w/Calcium (Tropicana®)
		Hot Cereal w/Low-Fat Milk & 1/2 Usual Amount of Sweetener
LUNCH	(3)	Fruit Salad
	(4)	Bran Muffins
	(5)	Frozen Juice on a Stick
DINNER	(6)	Cut Vegetable Salad w/Warm Tortillas
	(7)	Potato Soufflé
		Steamed Broccoli and Carrots
		Fresh Fruit Slices in Apricot Juice

DAY 3 - SUNDAY

Introduce more fresh fruits and fruit smoothies into your menu plan. Buy plastic or glass containers for bulk product storage. Reorganize your kitchen so that you feel comfortable with the new grains and legumes that will make up a large part of your diet. Look through the menus for the rest of the week and see if you can prepare any of the ingredients ahead of time to give yourself more time on busy weekdays.

BREAKFAST		Orange Juice w/Calcium
		Fearn® Pancakes w/Soy Milk
	(8)	Bananas & Strawberry Compote
		Herbal Tea
LUNCH	(9)	Sweet Potato Pancakes w/Applesauce
	(10)	Fruit Smoothie
DINNER	(11)	Burritos w/Refried Beans & Non-Fat Cheese
	(20)	Green Salad
	(12)	Salsa
	(13)	Guacamole

DAY 4 - MONDAY

Keep changes as simple as possible. Revise your child's lunchbox so that it has healthy finger foods (see Lunch for today). Let your children be on "demand feeding." If they want a snack before dinner, let them have it. I suggest fresh fruit, rice crackers, or cereal with soy milk. Cut dairy products from one meal. For example, substitute soy milk for cow's milk on breakfast cereal.

BREAKFAST (10)   Orange Juice Smoothie
                    Toast w/Fruit Conserve
                            (a jam with no additives
                            or added sugar)

LUNCHBOX   Carrot & Celery Sticks
         (14)   Bean Dip w/No-Oil Chips
                    Apple
                    Thermos of Water

DINNER   Mixed Green Salad w/Balsamic Vinegar
                    No-Oil Sourdough Rolls, Toasted
         (15)   Soup-Stew
         (16)   Fruit Cobbler

DAY 5 - TUESDAY

Center dinner around a big stir fry with rice or pasta. Add a new tofu dish to the meal. (see today's menu). Make a dip for vegetables. Continue to check your menus for the coming days. Eliminate egg yolks from your diet if you haven't already. Reduce your caffeine consumption, which means drinking less coffee and tea. Try herbal teas instead. Cut out soft drinks. Switch to carbonated water mixed with fruit juices.

BREAKFAST   Fresh Grapefruit and Orange Sections
Hot Cereal w/Soy Milk and Raisins

LUNCHBOX

Lettuce/Tomato/Avocado Sandwich
      w/ Mustard on Sourdough Roll
Japanese Seaweed Chips
      (health food store)
Apple

DINNER   (17)   Cut-Up Vegetables w/Lentil Dip
            (18)   Broiled Tamari Tofu
            (19)   Sautéed Leeks with Asparagus
                     (or Broccoli) w/Rice or Pasta
No-Oil Cookies w/Sliced Strawberries

DAY 6 - WEDNESDAY

Double check your kitchen to make certain you have only fat-free dairy products and whole grains on hand. Look ahead at the menus for the next seven days and begin to plan your shopping list for the week. At this stage, be very specific about which stores you need to go to for specific items. Make the health food store your first stop instead of the last.

BREAKFAST	Melon Slices
	Cereal w/Soy Milk and aTouch of
	Sweetener (if necessary)
	(Try soy milk with vanilla.
	It's a good substitute for
	sweeteners.)
LUNCHBOX	Almond Butter Sandwich onWhole
	Grain Bread w/slices of bananas
	Cut-up Vegetables
	Apple
	Mineral Water

DINNER	(20)	Green Salad w/Sprouts and Beans
	(21)	Pasta w/Tomato Sauce
		Toasted Sourdough Slices
	(22)	Bananas w/Fruit Sauce

DAY 7 - THURSDAY

Start thinking ecologically. Cut back on paper and plastic products. Use and reuse rags, canvas shopping bags cloth napkins and cloth diapers. Cut down on paper towel usage. Check detergents and cleaners to make sure they are as safe as possible for the environment. Buy as few canned and boxed products as possible. If you have a garden, think about setting aside space for compost.

BREAKFAST	(10)	Fruit Smoothie Toast w/Fruit Conserve
LUNCHBOX		Mixed Sprout Sandwich w/Lettuce, Tomato & Mustard on Whole Wheat Bread No-Oil Chips Apple Mineral Water
DINNER	(23) (24)	Corn and Bean Salad on Romaine Japanese Pasta w/Julienne Vegetables Rice Dream® Custard (A brand name product found in Health Food Stores)

DAY 8 - FRIDAY

Congratulations! This is the first day of Week Two of your family's new way of living. This is a good time to start a recipe journal to keep notations on the foods your family likes most. This can be on file cards, in a book, or on the computer. Put favorite recipes on cards on the refrigerator until you're comfortable making them. Look ahead to weekend plans.

BREAKFAST (10)   Soy Milk Smoothie w/Bananas
                   Black Bread Toast w/Honey

LUNCHBOX   Thermos of Soup
                   Leftover Corn & Bean Salad
                   Sourdough Bread
                   Dried Fruit

DINNER   (25)   Caesar Salad with Croutons
           (26)   Shish-Kebab with Tofu on Basmati Rice
                   Slices of Melon w/ Fresh Berries

DAY 9 - SATURDAY

After shopping, plan to bake bread. Let the children get involved. A bread machine is a wonderful investment if your family likes bread. Try being more innovative in your food choices. Cut dairy products out of a second meal so they are only being served once a day (if at all) and then serve only fat-free products. Make some Fruit Juice on a Stick treats for your children.

BREAKFAST		Glass of Fruit Juice
	(27)	Soy Milk Pancakes w/Fresh Fruit
LUNCH		Platter of Cut-Up Vegetables
		(Add some radishes and jicama.)
		with
	(28)	Tahini Dip
	(13)	Guacamole
DINNER	(29)	Cabbage Salad
	(30)	Hearty Bean Soup
	(31)	Homemade Baked Bread
		Fresh fruit

DAY 10 - SUNDAY

Plan a big breakfast or brunch around freshly-baked, whole-grain bran muffins. Plan for a dinner out at a restaurant where you can be sure they will serve vegetarian food. Italian is a great choice. Find a restaurant which does not use sulfites in their salads and where there is a no-smoking policy.

BREAKFAST		Fresh Fruit, Cut-Up
	(4)	Freshly Baked Muffins
		Cereal with Soy Milk
		Herbal Tea
LUNCH	(32)	Soy Cheese Pizza
		Apples
DINNER		Eat out! Eat wisely! Avoid
		fats and salty food. Don't be
		afraid to inquire about how
		foods are prepared and to
		ask for what you want when
		you order in a restaurant.

DAY 11 - MONDAY

Cut all flesh foods out of your diet, including chicken and fish. Keep an eye on your fat intake, and use only small amounts of oils. Raw foods should be a major part of your diet, so check to see that your refrigerator is full of fruits and vegetables. Keep some cut up and ready to snack.

BREAKFAST (31)   Homemade Baked Bread w/Honey
Fresh Fruit Slices

LUNCHBOX   Soy Pizza (leftover from Sunday)
Melon Slices

DINNER   (33)   Antipasto Salad
(34)   Stuffed Artichokes
Melon in season

DAY 12 - TUESDAY

Stock the refrigerator with cold pastas in fun shapes that the children can snack on easily. Cut back further on caffeine and other stimulants. All sodas should be gone by now. Try to get through one day without any dairy or egg white products. Set out a definite exercise plan, and decide as a family how to stick to it. This can be as simple as taking a walk together every day before dinner or doing 15 minutes of aerobics in the morning. Find what works best for you.

BREAKFAST	(10)	Apple Fruit Smoothie
	(4)	Bran Muffins
LUNCHBOX		No-Fat Cheese Sandwich
		Fresh Fruit
		Carbonated Water
DINNER	(35)	Marinated Salad
	(36)	"Pork and Beans"
	(37)	Baked Orange Slices

DAY 13 - WEDNESDAY

Plant an herb garden, either outdoors or on your kitchen windowsill. Begin to plan your meals for the next week. As a family, talk about which foods you'd like to have again in the next few days. Get input from everyone. Cut out cheese products, and keep your intake of all dairy products, including non-fat yogurt, to a minimum.

BREAKFAST   Fresh Fruit Juice
                 Cereal w/Soy Milk

LUNCHBOX   Thermos of Soup
        (4)   Bran Muffins
                 Fruit Juice

DINNER   (38)   Sprout Salad w/Sesame Dressing
         (39)   Clear Soup w/Mushrooms
         (40)   Stuffed Wontons
                 Fresh Fruit

DAY 14 - THURSDAY

You did it! You've changed your diet and your life! Now, finish planning your shopping list for the next week. Spend most of your food dollars in the health food or natural food store. Look for fruits and vegetables that are organically grown. Reflect on the ways your life has improved since your family's been on the new regimen.* Treat yourself to a couple of other vegetarian cookbooks so you can experiment and vary your menus to keep your family asking for more healthy foods.

BREAKFAST		Fresh Fruit
		Hot Cereal w/Chopped Dates
LUNCHBOX		Cut-Up Vegetables
	(4)	Bran Muffin
		No-Fat Cheese Stick
		Banana
		Mineral water
DINNER	(40)	Shredded Vegetable Salad
	(41)	Stir-Fry w/Tofu
	(42)	Rice Pudding

* Try not to be discouraged. Changes are not alway smooth or fun, and kids don't always adapt easily.

MEYERA'S RECIPES

MEYERA'S RECIPES

Unless otherwise stated, all of these recipes are designed to feed four adults. If your family is larger or if you want leftovers, simply double the amounts. The numbers next to the menu dishes listed in THE 14 DAY TRANSITION PLAN correspond to the recipes in this section of the book. If you have a very young child, be sure to look at the end of the recipe section. I have given you some ideas for preparing wonderfully nutritious homemade baby food. I have also included some suggestions for foods to put in school lunchboxes so you can keep these lunches interesting – and make sure they're eaten!

1. STIR-FRY VEGETABLES WITH BROWN RICE

2 c short grain brown rice
4 1/2 c cold water

In a saucepan, combine the rice and water. Bring to a boil.
Turn down heat to simmer and then cover, cooking for 35 minutes.
Turn off heat. Leave lid on and allow rice to stand for 20 minutes.

Meanwhile, prepare Stir-Fry.

2 tbsp olive oil
2 med size onions, chopped
2 cloves of garlic, chopped
1 inch piece of ginger, sliced lengthwise
3 carrots, cut into diagonal slices 1/8 inch thick
2 c chopped celery
1 c sliced mushrooms
1 small green pepper, sliced
1 small red pepper sliced
1 1/2 c sliced zucchini or yellow squash
1 c broccoli flowerettes*
1 to 2 tbsp soy sauce or tamari (Japanese soy sauce)

In a wok or skillet, heat the oil and add the next three ingredients. Stir and saute for 5 minutes. Next, add all remaining ingredients except for the soy sauce. Stir and cook for 8 more minutes. Add
the soy sauce and stir all vegetables to coat them. Cook for another 2
to 3 minutes. Serve hot over a bed of short grain brown rice. Top
with toasted sesame seeds.

*Green flower-like sections at the top of the stalk.

2. BAKED APPLES WITH STRAWBERRIES

4 organically-grown Granny Smith or Macintosh apples

Core the apples and place them standing up in a Pyrex® dish.

1 c water
2 tbsp honey
1/2 tsp cinnamon
sprinkle of ground cloves

In a saucepan, heat and combine the ingredients. Next, pour the mixture over the apples. Bake at 350° for 35 minutes. Remove and cool slightly. Serve with sliced strawberries and some of the liquid poured over the apples. Top with chopped nuts.

3. FRUIT SALAD

Although canned fruit salads are available, nothing tastes better than a mixture of your favorite fresh fruits. Cut up chunks of melons and berries, and add grapes. Toss in slices of kiwi, banana, and pineapple for a tropical flavor. Try not to use any sweetener. The fruit is naturally sweet enough.

Orange juice makes a good liquid for fruit salads. When possible, try to buy seasonal fruits. Sprinkle your salad with a little shredded coconut on top, chopped nuts, or add a refreshing mint leaf!

4. BRAN MUFFINS

Makes 8 to 10 muffins.

2 c unbleached flour
3 c bran
1 tsp baking powder
1 tsp soy oil
1 c soy milk
1/2 c apple juice
1 egg white (or an egg equivalent found in health food stores
   called Egg Replacer®)
1/4 c molasses
1/4 c brown sugar or honey
1/4 c raisins or 1/2 c seasonal fruit
   (Peaches, strawberries and blueberries are great!)

Preheat oven to 350° Combine first three ingredients in a
bowl and set aside. Combine all other ingredients and mix thoroughly. Add the dry ingredients to the wet ingredients and combine well,
but do not beat.

Line a muffin tin with paper cupcake liners and pour the batter evenly in each liner. Bake for 18 to 20 minutes (a little longer if
they are still wet). Let stand for 5 minutes and then remove the
muffins to a wire rack to cool.

You can prepare the batter the night before and refrigerate it,
but don't add the fruit until just before baking. Let the refrigerated
batter stand at room temperature for a 1/2 hour before baking.

5. FROZEN JUICE ON A STICK

You'll have to purchase molds at the store to make this treat which is similar to a Popsicle®. Fill the mold with 1/2 fruit juice and 1/2 water. For variety, add diced fresh fruit.

Try berries, peaches, or pineapple.

Fruit smoothies (see recipe 10) can also be poured into the molds and served frozen.

6. CUT VEGETABLE SALAD WITH WARM TORTILLAS

3 carrots, chopped
1 bunch of celery, chopped
1/4 head purple cabbage, chopped
1 yellow squash, coarsely grated
6 medium mushrooms, sliced
2 medium tomatoes, seeded* and chopped
1c broccoli flowerets with some stem, chopped
3 scallions, chopped (also called green onions)

Combine all of the above ingredients in a salad bowl.

1/3 c balsamic vinegar
1 tsp. granulated garlic or two cloves of minced fresh garlic
1 tsp. dried dillweed
a dash of ground pepper
1/4 c chopped parsley
1/4 c water

Mix the second group of ingredients together in a bowl with a whisk or shake well in a jar. Pour the dressing over the vegetables, and then toss the salad. Serve with warmed tortillas which can be eaten separately or wrapped around portions of the salad.

*To seed the tomatoes: cut them in half and scoop out all of the seeds, leaving as much of the tomato intact as possible.

7. POTATO SOUFFLÉ

Serves 6 to 8.

5 lbs baking potatoes

Wash and cube the potatoes. Cover them with water in a large pot and bring to a boil. Turn down the heat and simmer for about 20 minutes. You want them soft but not mushy.

Allow them to cool a little.

1 c vegetable broth
2 tbsp soy sauce or tamari
4 tsp granulated garlic
1 c soy milk

In a food processor, put some of the cooked potatoes, about 1 1/2 cups, and one quarter each of the above four ingredients. Blend well, but not too long otherwise the potatoes will get sticky. Repeat the process four times until all the potatoes are puréed. Fill a baking dish with the potato soufflé and top with bread crumbs. Bake uncovered for 40 minutes at 375°.

8. BANANA & STRAWBERRY COMPOTE

1/2 c puréed strawberries
1/2 c orange juice
2 tbsp honey
1 cinnamon stick
dash of nutmeg
1 c of sliced fresh strawberries
1 c of sliced bananas
1/4 c raisins
1/2 c wheatgerm (optional)

Combine the first five ingredients, and heat until the honey is melted. Add the fruit and raisins, and simmer for 6 to 8 minutes. Serve warm with some chopped nuts or wheat germ sprinkled on top.

9. SWEET POTATO PANCAKES WITH APPLE SAUCE

Makes 10 to 18 pancakes.

3 large sweet potatoes or yams
1/2 onion, grated
1/3 c whole wheat flour
1 egg white or egg replacer equivalent

Grate the potatoes and onions into a bowl. Add the flour and egg white, and combine. Batter should be firm enough to hold shape but not dry. If it is too wet, add a little more flour as needed. Use a non-stick griddle so you don't need oil. Form pancakes and heat until almost done. Turn pancakes over to brown other side.

APPLESAUCE

3 sweet apples, cut into small pieces
1/2 c water or apple juice
1/2 tsp. cinnamon

Heat in a saucepan for about 10 minutes and serve warm with pancakes.

10. MIXED FRUIT SMOOTHIES

In a blender, place:

    1 c apple juice
    1 banana
    1 pear, diced (no need to peel it)
    a dash of nutmeg

Blend until smooth, and pour into glasses.

Variations:
    1) Start with apricot, pineapple, or orange juice.
    2) Blend in fresh strawberries.
    3) Add blueberries and grapes.
    4) Try orange juice with fresh pineapple and bananas.
    5) Mix soy milk with bananas or berries and a dash of vanilla.
    6) Add some honey (if the fruit isn't sweet enough).
    7) Freeze leftover smoothie mixture in a popsicle® mold with a stick handle, and serve as a treat.

11. BURRITOS WITH REFRIED BEANS

REFRIED BEANS

Cover 2 c dried pinto or black beans with purified water, and soak them overnight in a cool place. In the morning, drain the water. Cover the beans with fresh water, and cook for 1 1/2 hours until they are soft. Drain beans, and save liquid for use in soups. This stock can be frozen in easy-to-thaw-and-use portions.

    2 tbsp. molasses
    1/4 c honey
    1/2 c tomato sauce
     cooked beans

In a saucepan, combine all the ingredients, including cooked beans. Heat, stirring constantly. If the beans begin sticking to the pan, scrape the bottom with a wooden spoon.*

When the beans are soft and the liquid has turned "saucy" (in about 8 to 10 minutes), remove from heat.

RICE

    2 c cooked short grain brown rice.

Prepare rice as in recipe #1.

Continues...

FILLING

1 tbsp soy oil
1 large onion, sliced thinly
2 carrots, cut into thin 2 inch strips or grated
4 stalks of celery cut into thin 2 inch strips
2 cloves of garlic, chopped
1 c tomato wedges
1/2 c red and green pepper slices (combined)
2 c zucchini or yellow squash or broccoli or mushrooms, all cut into thin strips
2 tbsp soy sauce or tamari
1c grated soy cheese

Heat oil in a wok or frying pan, and saute´ the onions until they are translucent. Then add all of the other vegetables and saute´ for 8 minutes. Add the soy sauce, mix well, and then turn off heat.

To assemble burritos:

Place a tortilla in your hand, and spread 3 tbsp of refried beans on tortilla. Add 1/4 to 1/3 c vegetables, top with rice, and fold over the tortilla. Place the finished tortilla in a rectangular Pyrex® baking dish. Continue filling the tortillas and placing them in the dish until you run out of vegetables. Top with grated soy cheese. Bake at 350° only for 10 minutes. You want the cheese to melt without the burritos drying out.

Serve with Salsa and Guacamole.

Continues...

12. SALSA

3 ripe tomatoes, chopped coarsely
1/4 c chopped cilantro
2 green onions, chopped
1 clove of garlic, chopped
1 c tomato juice

Combine and toss. This can sit in the refrigerator for a few days, but it will get spicier as it sits.

13. GUACAMOLE

2 avocados, seeded and peeled
1 tomato, sliced
1/4 c chopped onion
1 clove of garlic, chopped
dash of cayenne pepper
1 tbs. cilantro

Combine all the ingredients in a food processor.
Turn food processor on and off until mixture is smooth. To keep fresh, put in an airtight container or press Saran Wrap® to the surface of the guacamole so no air touches it.

Guacamole does not last long, but it is quick to make.

14. BEAN DIP

Cover 2 c dried pinto or black beans with purified water, and soak them overnight in a cool place. In the morning, drain the water. Cover the beans with fresh water, and cook for 1 1/2 hours until they are soft. Drain beans, and save liquid for use in soups. This stock can be frozen in easy-to-thaw-and-use portions.

> 2 tbsp. molasses
> 1/4 c honey
> 1/2 c tomato sauce
> cooked beans

In a saucepan, combine all the ingredients. Heat, stirring constantly. If the beans begin sticking to the pan, scrape the bottom with a wooden spoon. (Metal utensils may scratch the bottom of a no-stick pan. Use wooden utensils for cooking whenever possible.)

When the beans are soft and the liquid has turned "saucy" (in about 8 to 10 minutes), remove from heat.

Place refried beans in the blender with one chopped tomato and a dash of cayenne pepper. Blend until smooth.

Serve with no-oil chips or vegetable slices.

15. SOUP-STEW

This can serve as a basic recipe for either a thick soup or a stew. You can vary it to add diversity to your menu and to accommodate what's in your refrigerator on any given day. I always make more than I need and freeze some. When put through a blender, it can become a sauce or a dip for chips.

Here are the basics:

3 onions, chopped
6 carrots, diced
1 bunch of celery, chopped (include leaves)
1 c chopped potato, unpeeled
1 parsnip, whole
2 tomatoes, chopped
4 cloves of garlic, chopped
2 tbsp soy sauce
2 tbsp sherry
2 zucchini, cut in 1/2 inch pieces
2 yellow squash, cut in 1/2 inch pieces
1 c cauliflower, chopped
1/2 c green pepper, chopped
1/2 c red pepper, chopped
1 bay leaf
1/2 bunch parsley
fresh dill or 2 tbsp dried dill weed

Simmer all of the above ingredients for 1 1/2 hours. Remove the parsnip and the bunch of parsley. Serve hot with a big piece of bread.

16. FRUIT COBBLER

Preheat oven to 350°.

6 washed, sliced peaches or pears (with skins)
1/3 c unbleached flour
1 tsp. cinnamon
dash of nutmeg
1/2 c orange juice
1/3 c honey
2 tbsp arrowroot dissolved in 1/4 c cold water

Combine the first four ingredients in a bowl and toss together. Pour into a baking dish. In a saucepan, combine the last three ingredients and heat until the honey is dissolved.

Pour over the fruit. Bake uncovered for 35 minutes at 350°. Top with chopped nuts or no oil granola. Serve warm.

17. LENTIL DIP

Makes 2 1/2 cups.

1 c green or red lentils
3 c purified water

Cook the ingredients in a saucepan for about 20 minutes until the lentils are soft. Drain off the excess water, and reserve it for use later in soups, etc.

1/2 tbsp canola oil
1/2 onion, chopped
2 cloves of garlic, minced
1 1/2C chopped tomato
1 tsp soy sauce or tamari
1 tsp thyme
dash of cayenne or Tabasco®

Heat oil. Add onions and garlic, and cook until onions are translucent. Add tomatoes, and sauté for 5 more minutes.

Add the rest of the ingredients, stir well, and turn off heat. Allow to cool slightly.

In a food processor, combine the lentils and the onion mix.

Purée until smooth. This recipe can be doubled and will keep well in the refrigerator for 4 to 5 days covered.

18.   BROILED TAMARI TOFU

1/4 c soy sauce
1/4 c water
1 tsp granulated garlic
1/4 c chopped scallions
1 lb extra firm tofu

Combine the first four ingredients in a bowl. Cut a 1 pound package of Extra Firm Tofu into strips (approx. 3 inches long, 1/2 inch wide, and 1/4 inch thick).

Dredge the slices in the soy marinade for a minute or two, coating all the tofu slices. Place the tofu on a cookie sheet, and broil for 3 to 5 minutes.

Turn the slices over, and broil an additional 3 to 5 minutes. If you want them crispy, broil them longer. Watch carefully so they don't burn.

Serve hot.

Makes a great snack!

19. SAUTÉED LEEKS

Prepare 2c cooked short grain brown rice as in Recipe 1 or make Basmati rice which is an Indian white or brown grain with a nutty flavor.

SAUTÉED LEEKS

2 tbsp olive oil
4 leeks, washed & chopped
   (use white parts only)
1 onions, chopped
1 clove garlic, chopped
1 yellow pepper, sliced thinly
1 c of sliced mushrooms
1 lb broccoli flowerets or asparagus spears
1 tbsp soy sauce
2 tbsp sherry
1 tbsp raw sesame seeds

Heat the oil and sauté the next three ingredients until the onions are translucent. Add the next three ingredients and sauté for 5 more minutes. Add the soy sauce and sherry, and combine all of the vegetables well. Cook for 3 more minutes.

Serve hot over a bed of rice and top with sesame seeds.

20.　GREEN SALAD WITH SPROUTS

Salads are a special part of any meal, and you can vary them endlessly. There are a number of new lettuces, cabbages, and wild greens available in the market. For example, you can find dandelion and wild mustard greens, lambs lettuce, bib, red romaine and green romaine, red leaf and green leaf, red butter lettuce, arugala (which is high in calcium), raddichio, and green and red cabbages.

Experiment with interesting vinegars like balsamic, blueberry, raspberry, wine, tarragon, cider, and rice vinegar.

You only need to use a hint of oil. Learn to eat greens for their own taste, and use less dressing.

Garnish with sprouts! There are many kinds of sprouts, and they are easy to grow. Here's how: use a jar with a wide neck, put 1/2 c lentils (or mung beans, alfalfa seeds, or sunflower seeds) in the jar, and cover with purified water. Cut a piece of cheese cloth to fit generously over the jar's neck, and secure it with a rubber band. Let the beans or seeds soak for 1hour, then pour out the water through the cheese cloth.

Shake the jar gently to distribute the seeds as evenly as possible, and let the jar sit on its side in a shady place.

We like to keep them out on the kitchen counter, near the sink – but out of the direct sun. Wet the seeds, and pour out the water 3 or 4 times a day. You don't have to soak them again. Some beans sprout in 48 hours; some take a few more days.

When the sprouts have little green tips, eat them! Put them in a container in the refrigerator. They will last 5 days.

21. PASTA WITH TOMATO SAUCE

Choose an interesting pasta so the kids will enjoy the meal. Now let's make a healthy sauce.

2 carrots, chopped
4 stalks of celery , chopped
1 onion, sliced

Cover the ingredients with purified water, and bring to a boil. Simmer for 15 minutes. Remove from the heat, and cool slightly. Drain the vegetables, reserving the liquid, and purée in the blender. (You can save the liquid, freeze it, and add it to soup later.) If you have tomato sauce made, just add the vegetable purée. If you need to make tomato sauce, here's a basic recipe.

4 lbs Italian plum tomatoes, chopped
1 large can tomato paste
1/2 c purified water
1 tbsp basil leaves
1 bay leaf
1/2 tbsp oregano
1 tsp granulated garlic

Combine all ingredients and simmer for 1 hour. Stirring occasionally so the sauce doesn't stick to the pot. Keep the heat low. When the sauce is done, you can add the vegetable purée mixture. Serve over pasta.

(Note: This is a great way to get more vitamins and minerals into the kids, and this dish tastes terrific!)

22. BANANAS WITH FRUIT SAUCE

1 c fresh strawberries or 1/2 c raspberries
1 tbsp soy milk
1/2 tsp vanilla
2 bananas, sliced

Purée the first three ingredients in the blender or food processor the first 3 ingredients. Arrange the banana slices in a circle and pour the purée over them. Top with a mint leaf.

23. CORN AND BEAN SALAD

1 c cooked black beans
1 c corn kernels
1/4 c chopped red pepper
1/4 c chopped green pepper
1/2 c grated carrot
1/2 c chopped celery
1/4 c chopped green onion
1/3 c balsamic vinegar
2 cloves garlic, chopped
1/4 c chopped parsley
1 tbsp dill weed
1/2 tsp. soy sauce

Prepare black beans. Drain off liquid. Combine first seven ingredients gently. In a bowl, whisk together the remaining ingredients, and then gently combine the dressing with the vegetables.

Clean romaine lettuce leaves, and arrange them on a plate to form a nest. Spoon out salad, and serve chilled.

24. JAPANESE PASTA WITH JULIENNED VEGETABLES

Buy soba noodles, which are available in most markets and health food stores in the oriental food section. They have a subtle taste and make a nice change from more familiar pastas. Cook according to directions on package.

To julienne vegetables, cut them in long, thin strips about 2 1/2 inches long.

    1 tsp sesame oil
    1 tbsp soy oil
    1 1/2 c sliced onions
    1/2 c green onions
    2 cloves garlic, minced
    1 1/2 c julienned carrots
    1 1/2 c julienned celery
    1 c sliced mushrooms
    1 c red or green (or mixed) julienned peppers
    1 c broccoli flowerettes
    1 1/2 tbsp soy sauce
    dash of cayenne
    1/4 c peanut sauce*
    1/2 c water

Heat oil and sauté the next three ingredients for 8 minutes. Then add the carrots and celery and sauté for three more minutes. Add the remaining vegetables. Toss well and continue cooking. Then add the soy sauce, cayenne, peanut sauce, and water. Stir well. Cook for five more minutes and remove from heat.

Portion out noodles on plates, and top with vegetables. Toasted sesame seeds are a tasty garnish.

*Can be purchased in health food stores.

25. CAESAR SALAD WITH CROUTONS

Chop and then chill romaine lettuce. Toast whole wheat bread, and let it stand for 10 minutes.

Cut toast into cubes.

DRESSING

In a jar, mix and shake well:

2 tsp olive oil
2 cloves garlic, crushed
1/4 c lemon juice
1 tbsp soy sauce
2 tbsp soy milk

Toss dressing with lettuce, and add croutons and a small amount of grated soy cheese.

26. SHISH KEBAB WITH TOFU ON BASMATI RICE

Prepare Basmati rice.

2 tbsp soy sauce
1/4 c dry sherry
4 cloves of garlic, pressed or minced
3 green onions, chopped finely
1/4 c peanut sauce or honey
1/2 c purified water
2 c extra firm tofu, cubed into 1 inch cubes
   (large enough to run a skewer through them)

In a bowl, stir together all the ingredients except the tofu. When combined well, gently toss the tofu, and let it sit in the marinade while you prepare the other vegetables.

1 red pepper, cut into wide strips
1 green pepper, cut into wide strips
2 carrots, cut into rounds 1/4 inch thick
1 c pearl onions
1 lb button mushrooms
1 1/2 c cherry tomatoes

Remove tofu from marinade with a slotted spoon, and place in a bowl. Toss all the other vegetables gently in the marinade.

Continues...

Take skewers or sticks and spear vegetables and tofu in a colorful order. For instance, try onion, tofu, tomato, green pepper, carrot, green pepper, tofu, and a mushroom. Place all the spears into a baking dish, and pour the marinade over them. Turn the skewers several times to wet all of the vegetables.

Barbecue the skewers, grill them on a home grill, or broil them in the oven until brown and cooked.

Serve on Basmati Rice. For a dipping sauce, you can select one of the many soy-based sauces or Gorilla barbecue sauce from the health food store.

27. SOY PANCAKES

Makes 8 pancakes.

1/4c whole wheat flour
1/4c buckwheat flour
1/2c unbleached flour
1/2 tsp. baking powder (aluminum-free)

Combine dry ingredients in a bowl. Slowly add: 1C soy milk plus with vanilla.

Keep mixing, or blend in blender until smooth. Sometimes I add an egg white, but I don't find it to be essential.

Drop large spoonfuls onto a greased skillet. When bubbles appear on top, flip it over for a few seconds and then transfer pancakes to a platter.

Serve with fresh fruit and fruit purées.

NOTE: To make crepes, use 1/8 - 1/4C more liquid.

For dinner crepes, use the soy milk <u>without</u> vanilla and make sure they are <u>cool</u> before stacking them.

For dessert crepes, use the soy milk with vanilla for a sweeter taste.

28. GREEN TAHINI

Combine in a blender:

1/2c tahini
1 tbs. lemon juice
1 tsp. tamari
pinch of cayenne pepper
1/4 - 1/2c water

When the tahini spread is smooth, add in the blender:

1/4c chopped arugola leaves
1/4c chopped parsley
1/2c chopped spinach

Blend together. This is a tasty sandwich spread that can be used with lettuce, tomato, cucumber, and sprouts.

29. CABBAGE SALAD

Serves 4 - 6.

2c red cabbage, shredded
3c green cabbage, shredded
1c grated carrots
1c chopped celery
1/4c chopped green onions
1 1/2c mung bean sprouts

Combine all the vegetables, and toss gently. In a separate bowl, whisk together the dressing.

1/4c water
1/2c red wine vinegar
1/4c dry sherry
2 tbsp honey
2 cloves garlic, minced
1/2 tsp soy sauce
1 tsp dried dill weed

Pour the dressing over the vegetables, and serve chilled on a bed of romaine lettuce or a large fresh cabbage leaf.

Note: This salad is wonderful as filling for a sandwich in a "hero roll" with grated soy cheese and soy bologna.

30. HEARTY BEAN SOUP   *Serves 6 to 8.*

The night before, soak 2 c white beans in a large saucepan in a cool place. The next morning, drain the water and fill the pot with fresh water. Cook for 1 1/2 hours until beans are tender. Save the liquid.

2 onions, chopped
3 carrots, chopped
2 c chopped celery
3 cloves of garlic, chopped
1 large ripe tomatoe, chopped
1 parsnip, washed and whole
2 potatoes, chopped with the skins on
3 c vegetable stock
1 c bean broth
1/4 c parsley, chopped
1 tbsp chervil
Soy sauce to taste
1/2 tsp black pepper
1 bay leaf

Combine all ingredients and cover w/water. Cook for 1 hour. Remove the parsnip, add the cooked beans, and continue cooking for another hour. If you need more liquid, add some bean broth or boiling water. Serve hot with warm bread. This is a hearty soup and can be considered the main dish of your meal!

31. HOMEMADE WHOLE WHEAT BREAD

Makes 2 loaves.

In a small bowl, mix:

1/2 c warm (not hot!) water
1 package of dried yeast
1 tsp maple syrup or honey

Stir gently, then cover and place in warm area (such as the inside of an unlighted gas oven).

In another bowl, combine:

1/3 c water
1 tbsp soy oil
1 tbsp soy sauce

In a large bowl, sift together:

2 c white flour
1 1/4 c whole wheat flour

Add to the flour bowl:

1/4 c sunflower seeds
4 tbsp bran
3 tbsp oats
2 tbsp red wheat flakes (from health food store)

Make a well in the center of the dry ingredients, and add the wet ingredients – including the yeast mixture. Mix until all is combined. Knead for 15 minutes, turning the dough towards the center. Place the dough in a greased bowl. Cover and let stand in a warm place for 1 hour. (An unlighted gas oven is good for this step as well.)

Remove the dough, which will be doubled in size. Punch it down and knead on a floured board for 15 minutes more.

Divide the bread dough into 2 loaves, mold them into shape and place them on a greased baking sheet. Cover and let stand for 1 hour.

Bake at 375° for 40 to 45 minutes, until the bread sounds hollow when tapped on the bottom.

Allow the loaves to cool before slicing.

32. SOY CHEESE PIZZA

You can buy pizza dough or pizza pie shells, but here's my recipe. Then add your own vegetable tomato sauce, the kids' favorite vegetables, and top with grated soy cheese. Bake until the cheese is browned.

Pizza Dough Recipe:

1 pkg dry yeast
1 1/3 c warm (not hot) water
pinch of sugar
2 tbsp olive oil
dash of salt
2c sifted flour
1c whole wheat flour

Combine the yeast, water, and pinch of sugar in a bowl. Cover and let stand in a warm place (the inside of an unlit gas oven is usually 85°).

Sift the flours together. When the yeast rises, add the rest of the ingredients and yeast mix to the flours. Knead for about 10 minutes, and let rise once, covered in a warm place for about 2 hours.

Lightly oil 2 pizza pie pans 12 inch diameter or a cookie sheet. When the dough is ready, put it down and stretch it out to fill the pans. Pinch up the edges to form a little wall to hold the sauce and vegetables. Prick the dough with a fork several times.

Spread sauce and vegetables and top with grated soy cheese. Bake at 400° for about 1/2 hour.

33. ANTIPASTO SALAD

Everybody likes to pick and taste, so here's an opportunity to treat the family to a fun appetizer. It may seem like work at first, but after a while you can serve leftovers plus condiments. For example, an antipasto might consist of:

carrot and celery sticks
artichoke hearts or quartered freshly cooked artichokes
marinated roasted peppers*
cherry tomatoes
avocado slices
cold, cooked asparagus spears
marinated mushrooms and eggplant cubes*
marinated broccoli and cauliflower*
soy cheese slices
soy bologna slices
bean dip

Arrange on a large platter, and garnish with parsley. Serve with toasted sourdough bread.

* Recipes on next page

*MARINATED ROASTED PEPPERS

Before marinating the peppers, core and seed them. Then, roast the peppers on an open flame on the stove – or under the broiler – until charred. Let cool and then peel off all burnt skins which are great for compost. Slice the peppers in eighths, and marinate in balsamic vinegar for 1/2 hour. Refrigerate covered. The peppers will keep for several days. They're also great chopped up in salad.

*MARINATED MUSHROOMS AND EGGPLANT CUBES

To make a warm marinade for the mushrooms and egg-plant cubes (or broccoli and cauliflower), place the following ingredients in a frying pan:

1 c water
6 peppercorns
3 cloves of garlic, sliced
1/2 c dry sherry
1 tbsp soy sauce (optional)
1/4 c lemon juice
1 bay leaf
1/2 piece of fresh ginger (optional)

Bring to a boil, and then turn down the heat. Add the veg-etables – a few at a time – and simmer for 6 to 10 minutes. Do not overcook. Remove the vegetables with a slotted spoon and refrigerate. (The vegetables are also a great snack with crackers.)

34. STUFFED ARTICHOKES

Take 4 firm, bright green artichokes. Trim the sharp points off the tips of the leaves and cut off the stems so the chokes can sit up.

Bring a large pot of water to a boil. (Artichokes like room to move.) Add 1/4 c lemon juice or squeeze in juice of 2 fresh lemons. This keeps the chokes from turning dark while they cook. Boil the artichokes for 35 minutes. You do not want to overcook them. Take a table knife and gently stab one through the bottom. If it is easy to do, then they are ready. Remove the artichokes carefully, turning them upside down to drain and cool.

In the meantime, prepare the filling. Put 1 tbsp olive oil in a frying pan, and add:

> 1/2 c chopped green onions
> 1/2 c chopped celery
> 4 cloves of garlic, minced

Sauté for 5 minutes. Then add:

> 1 1/2 cups sliced mushrooms
> 1 c firm tofu, cut into small cubes
> 1 tbsp soy sauce

Add:
3/4 c bread crumbs

Toss until well mixed.

Now back to the artichokes. Carefully open the top of each choke so you can get down to the center and remove the prickly leaves that surround the heart. I use a grapefruit spoon to scrape them out, being careful not to disturb the tender heart meat. When the inside of the choke is empty, add enough filling to come to the top and then sit the choke in a baking dish. Repeat with the other chokes and then bake at 350° for 15 minutes. No longer – you don't want them to dry out!

Now serve. (I open up the artichoke and eat some leaf and some filling at the same time. That way, I don't miss the taste of oily sauces!)

35. MARINATED SALAD

1 c grated carrots
1 c chopped celery
1 c cauliflower pieces
1/2 c chopped green onions
1 c sliced mushrooms
1 1/2 c chopped red cabbage
1/2 c chopped jicama or sliced water chestnuts

Prepare all the vegetables, and combine in a salad bowl. Set aside, and whisk together the dressing ingredients:

1/4 c balsamic vinegar
2 tsp minced garlic
1 tsp dried dill weed
2 tbsp water
2 tbsp chopped parsley

Pour the dressing over the salad, and gently toss. Garnish with tomato wedges and your favorite sprouts.
Sometimes I grate soy cheese and top the salad with it!

36. "PORK" AND BEANS

In the health food stores, and now in many supermarkets, you can find an assortment of soy "hot dogs."

Try several brands, and choose your family's favorite for this dish.

Split the franks lengthwise and place them on the grill or griddle to cook. Heat until they are cooked through – about 10 minutes. Set aside.

Prepare red kidney beans. In a frying pan add:

3c beans, cooked
1 onion, chopped
1 clove of garlic, minced
1 tomato, chopped

Cook over low heat, scraping the bottom of the pan so the beans don't stick.

Cut the franks into 1 inch pieces and add to bean mixture. Serve hot.

37. BAKED ORANGE SLICES

In a saucepan, mix:

1/2 c orange juice
1/2 c apple juice
2 tbsp honey
1/4 c raisins
dash of cinnamon
dash of nutmeg

Let simmer until honey is melted (about 3 minutes). Set aside.

Peel 2 or 3 oranges, and slice them into quarters. Place orange slices in a small baking dish, and pour sauce over them. Broil for 6 to 8 minutes. Watch closely! You don't want the slices to burn, but the sauce should thicken slightly.

Serve hot.

38. SESAME DRESSING

In a jar, mix the following ingredients and shake well:

1 tbsp sesame oil
1 tbsp soy oil
4 tbsp rice vinegar
1 tbsp dry sherry (optional)
1/2 tsp granulated garlic
dash of soy sauce
1 tbsp honey
2 tbsp water

Pour over a mixture of sprouts and shredded lettuce.

39. CLEAR SOUP WITH MUSHROOMS

Serves 4 to 6.

Wash and cut stems off of 2 ounces of Chinese dried black mushrooms. Pour 2 c boiling water over them, and let them sit for 1/2 hour. Drain and reserve liquid. Cut the mushrooms into slices. Set aside.

Meanwhile, in a large pot, combine:

2 onions, cut in quarters
3 scallions, whole
1 to 2 inch piece of ginger, cut in half lengthwise
2 carrots, washed & whole
4 stalks of celery , whole
4 sprigs of parsley
1 sprig of fresh dill
2 garlic cloves, cut in half
3 c whole button mushrooms

Add enough water to cover, plus 3 c more. Bring to a boil. Turn down heat and simmer, partially covered, for 2 hours. Then remove the lid, and carefully strain the liquid into another pot. To the clear liquid, add the black mushrooms with:

1 tbsp soy sauce
1/2 tsp white ground pepper
1/2 c chopped scallions
1/4 c dry sherry
1/2 tsp sesame oil (optional)

Simmer for 30 minutes longer, and serve with brown rice or noodles.

40. STUFFED WONTONS   *Makes 30 wontons.*

Buy wonton skins at your local market. Read the labels carefully. Look for packaged wontons without additives.

Filling:

1 tsp sesame oil
1 tsp soy oil
1 to 2 inch piece of ginger, sliced lengthwise
1 onion, chopped
2 carrots, grated
1/2 c chopped celery
1 c grated mushrooms
1 tbsp soy sauce
1/2 c bread crumbs

Heat oil in a wok or skillet and add the next four ingredients.
Stir-fry for 6 minutes. Add the mushrooms and continue cooking for
another 2 minutes, then add the soy sauce. Turn off heat and spoon
vegetables into a bowl. Add the bread crumbs, and mix well. Set
aside,and allow to cool for a half hour.

To assemble, have a small bowl of water handy. Lay out a wonton skin, and spoon 1 tsp of filling into the center. Dip a *clean* finger
into the water, and wet 2 adjacent edges of the wonton skin. Fold the
other 2 edges over to form a triangle shape, and press them together.
Place on a baking sheet. You can do this assembly-line fashion, wet-
ting each one just before you fold it over.

Set up a steamer. Lightly oil the basket, and steam wontons for
2 minutes. Serve with peanut sauce or soy sauce. These can be
made the day before and sealed with plastic wrap in the refrigerator.

41. SHREDDED VEGETABLE SALAD

Try this variation on a theme!

Shred zucchini, broccoli (lightly steamed), anf carrots, and slice mushrooms. Add to chopped celery. The quantities aren't important. Use more of whatever your family likes.

Toss with a flavorful vinegar mixed with a little honey and a dash of sherry. Rice vinegar is great here, topped with toasted sesame seeds and sprouts. Or add sunflower seeds instead, and serve on Boston lettuce.

This leftover salad marinates well and will taste great at lunch the next day.

42. STIR FRY WITH TOFU

Heat a wok or skillet for a minute or two. Add:

1 tbsp sesame oil
1 tbsp soy oil
2 cut up onions
2 julienned carrots
a 2 inch slice of ginger, cut lengthwise
3 cloves of garlic, minced
1/2 c green onions, chopped

Sauté for 8 minutes, and then add:

1 c sliced mushrooms
1 1/2 c firm tofu, diced
2 oz prepared black mushrooms
1 can sliced water chestnuts
1 head of bok choy, washed well & sliced

Sauté for another 5 minutes, and add:

2 c mung bean sprouts
1 to 2 tbsp soy sauce
1/4 c dry sherry or rice wine

Simmer for 3 minutes more, and serve hot on a bed of short grain brown rice.

43. RICE PUDDING

Prepare brown rice to yield 2 1/2 cups cooked.

2 1/2 c soy milk
2 tbsp honey
2 tbsp molasses
1 tsp vanilla
2 tbsp agàr-agar flakes (a natural gelling agent that
        comes from seaweed and is found in health food
        stores)

Combine all ingredients except rice in a saucepan and bring
to a boil stirring. Turn down heat, and simmer until thick (just
a few minutes) Then add:

1 tsp orange juice
1/2 c dates or raisins

In a baking dish, spread out the cooked rice and pour the
soy milk mixture over it. Bake at 350° for about an hour. You
may top this with no-oil cookie crumbs.
Great served hot or cold!

BABY FOOD

The first step is to buy a mini-processor. Then you can:

Mash a banana.

Mash a pear, and add a little peeled apple.

Mash cooked sweet potatoes or cooked
organic carrots. Mash potatoes with soy milk.

Mash cooked broccoli, add a few cooked
peas. Puree´ cooked rice with soy milk.

When preparing baby foods, there's no need to season anything. Allow your children to become accustomed to the "real"
taste of foods. Some they'll like; some they'll reject. It's not
necessary to be creative for 6 to 12-month-old children. Most
are perfectly happy with the basic tastes of food.

When you mash cooked white potatoes, add a little soy
milk or non-fat, plain yogurt if the potatoes need some liquid.
Never add milk or butter!

Fruits and vegetables are the first foods you should introduce. Be careful with strawberries, blueberries, and tomatoes.
Many children are allergic or sensitive to them. Start with
bananas. Later, you can add mashed potatoes, squash, broccoli,
sweet potatoes and peas.

When your child is 9 to 12 months-old, start taking any
soup you are making and separate a portion of it before you
add the seasonings. Puree the bland soup. If the vegetable
tastes are too strong, dilute with water, but not with too much.

Thicker soups are usually accepted more easily by very young children.

Blend smoothies. (See Recipe 10 for adult version)

For example,
1) apple juice, water, and fresh pears;
2) apple juice, water, and fresh peaches;
3) apple juice, soy milk, and banana; or
4) Pear juice, banana and soy milk.,

These smoothies can be thinned with water or fed to a baby as part of any meal.

SCHOOL LUNCHES

Here's a real mind-bender. There is no easy solution to the challenge of what to send to school for your child to eat. However, I do have some hints that may help.

√   Don't use mayonnaise on a sandwich. Instead, use a touch of mustard.

√   Use almond butter instead of peanut butter.

√   In place of jelly, use sugarless "spreadable fruit" conserve. Be sparing even with these. The sweet taste will help form early habits that can be hard to break.

√   Add slices of banana or apple to an almond butter sandwich.

√   Grow sprouts at home and make lettuce, tomato, and sprout sandwiches on whole-wheat bread or a roll with a touch of mustard.

√   Send carrot and celery sticks with a small container of yogurt dip, bean dip or guacamole´.

√   Always pack fruit. Even better, pack several small pieces of different fruits for variety.

√   Make a "hero" sandwich. I usually slice the bread and put mustard on it. Then I seal it in plastic wrap. In a baggie, I put lettuce, tomato, and sprouts, along with a cut-up pickle. When Simone is in school, she can assemble the sandwich herself. It tastes fresh, and the bread isn't soggy.

√   Pack a container of left-over pastas in fun shapes. Kids love it.

√   Avoid the hot school lunches. They're often greasy, sugary, and full of animal products.

√   Our local public school has a salad bar. It's not great, but it's better than the hot lunch. If your school district has a salad bar, encourage your children to enjoy fresh greens at lunch.

√   Pack in small reusable plastic containers a variety of tasty treats plus fresh fruit.

GLOSSARY

Carcinogen: Any agent or substance which has been shown to cause cancer under certain conditions.

Cholesterol: A waxy substance manufactured and used by the body to build cell walls and produce vitamin D and bile acids. Our bodies produce enough cholesterol for our needs. If we eat excess amounts, cholesterol begins to build up in the arteries and forms plaque which blocks the flow of blood and leads to strokes and heart attacks. It is advisable that your overall cholesterol level be under 200, preferably in the 150 to 170 range.

Cholesterol readings are often broken down into two different types, *HDL Cholesterol* and *LDL Cholesterol* (sometimes referred to as Good Cholesterol and Bad Cholesterol).

Higher levels of HDL (high-density lipoprotein) cholesterol mean you are metabolizing cholesterol faster than people with lower levels. Your HDL level should be above 35 mg/dl.

LDL (low-density lipoprotein) cholesterol is the most damaging to the walls of the arteries. High LDL levels can be indicators of heart disease. Your LDL Cholesterol level should be below 130 mg/dl.

There is also a distinction that should be made between *Blood Cholesterol* and *Dietary Cholesterol*. *Blood Cholesterol* is also known as serum cholesterol. This is the reading you get when you have a blood test. *Dietary Cholesterol* refers to the cholesterol that you eat in foods.

Diverticulosis: A pouchlike bulging through the muscular layer of the large intestine (colon), particularly in the sigmoid colon which is above the rectum.

Electrolytes: An element or compound that, when melted or dissolved in water or other solvent, breaks up into ions and is able to carry an electric current. The body must have the correct amounts of the main electrolytes to use energy.

Fats: Body substances, composed of carbon, hydrogen. and small amounts of oxygen, that are not water-soluble. Fat contains more energy and calories than carbohydrates and proteins. (One gram of fat equals nine calories even though one gram of carbohydrate or protein equals only four calories.) The different types of fat are the result of varied bonding of the carbon, hydrogen and oxygen atoms.

Glycerol: The framework of linked carbon atoms which forms the basic structure of all fats. When three fatty acids are added to this framework, the structure becomes known as a *triglyceride*.

Saturated Fat: When all the hydrogen atoms are present in the fatty acid structure, it's called saturated. Animal fats, coconut, chocolate, hydrogenated oils, and palm oils, are all high in saturated fatty acids. These fats tend to raise cholesterol levels and have been linked to a large number of diseases, from atheroschlerosis to cancer.

Monounsaturated Fat: When one pair of hydrogen atoms is missing, as in avocados and olive oil, the structure is known as a monounsaturated fatty acid. Touted as the "good fat," it is still wise to keep consumption low.

207

Polyunsaturated Fat: In this form of fatty acid, at least two pairs of hydrogen atoms are missing. Most vegetable oils (especially safflower and sunflower) and fish oils fall into this group. While polyunsaturated fats have been shown to reduce atherosclerosis, they have also been linked to increased incidences of colon cancer.

Fiber: Any substance in plant foods that is not digested. Fiber doesn't contribute to our growth, and it is possible to sustain life without it. However, fiber does contribute to the overall health of the body.

Water-insoluble fiber comes primarily from wheat brans and whole wheat, and also from the skins of fruit and vegetables. Cellulose, hemicellulose, and lignin are all insoluble fibers. In the body, these fibers soak up water and provide bulk to the stool so the fecal matter moves more quickly through the intestine. This decreases the incidence of constipation, colon cancer, diverticulosis, and other intestinal diseases.

Water soluble fiber is found in grains, legumes, fruits, and vegetables. They include pectin and the various gums that are extracted and added to processed foods. The water soluble fibers are thought to be very helpful in lowering blood cholesterol and decreasing blood lipids. In this way, they are instrumental in preventing or reversing heart disease.

Free Radicals: These are chemical compounds created in foods. The *free radical* is short one electron so it scavenges or steals an electron from tissue in the body. This creates a domino effect of tissue destruction which causes premature aging of everything from the heart muscle to skin cells. These unstable oxygen molecules, which can be the result of grilling meat over hot coals, are also a known carcinogen.

Fructose: The sweetest of all natural sweeteners, this monosaccharide (simple) sugar is derived from fruit. It is about 70% sweeter than more commonly used sucrose and in large quantities can cause abdominal pain and diarrhea.

Glucose: This is a monosaccharide (simple) sugar, which is also known as *dextrose.* Glucose is only two-thirds as sweet as sucrose.

Hydrogenated: To combine with hydrogen or to reduce with hydrogen.

Lactase: Natural enzyme is the human intestine that allows us to digest lactose. With age, the production of lactase decreases causing many people to have trouble digesting dairy products.

Lactose: A disaccharide sugar found in cow's milk which is a combination of glucose and galactose.

Legumes: These beans and peas, including kidney beans, pinto beans, soybeans, chickpeas, lentils, split peas, and peanuts, are the best sources of vegetable protein. When served with any grain or cereal food, the amino-acid balance becomes an acceptable substitute for meat protein.

Lipids: Basically lipids and fats are synonymous, although lipids include hormones, cholesterol, and wax.

Nitrates/Nitrites: Agents added to processed foods to inhibit the growth of botulism-causing bacteria. Nitrates and nitrites are commonly found in processed meats, most prominently bacon. These substances can become carcinogenic as they are cooked or digested. They should be avoided.

Organic Foods: and vitamins – Popularly, this refers to any food grown without the use of chemical fertilizers or pesticides.

PCB: Poly-Chlorinated Biphenyls are highly pollutant chemicals which were used widely in industrial products and processes beginning in the 1930s. Today, they are banned but they are stored in body fat and PCB residue can still be detected in breast milk and commercial foods. The American Academy of Pediatrics has stated that women do not need to fear breast feeding unless they have been exposed to PCB's at work or have eaten large amounts of freshwater fish from polluted lakes.

PKU: Phenylketonuria is a rare, hereditary metabolic disorder causing an inability to oxidize phenylalanine (an amino acid needed for growth in children and for processing protein throughout life). PKU patients should not be given aspartame or any derivative product.

Plaque: Waxy build-up on the inside walls of the arteries which restricts the blood flow and increases the likelihood of strokes and heart attacks.

Sucrose: This is a disaccharide (double molecule) sugar derived from sugar cane and beets. Sucrose – a combination of fructose and glucose (dextrose) – includes products such as raw sugar, turbinado (partially refined sugar), refined white table sugar, and brown and confectioner sugars.

Sulfites: Preservatives used on seafood, meat, vegetables, and dried fruits to preserve color and freshness. Also found in wines, sulfites must now be listed on the ingredient label. It's estimated that more than one million Americans are highly sensitive to these preservatives with reactions ranging from shortness of breath and hives to unconsciousness and, in extreme cases, death.

Triglycerides: These are the fats which are floating in your blood. If you were to have your blood tested right after eating a high fat meal, and the blood were left in a test tube for several hours, these fats would rise to the top of the tube. High triglyceride levels can lead to heart attacks, diabetes, and poor circulation. High triglyceride levels, those over 200 mg/dl, can be caused by fats in the diet and by simple sugars, including fresh fruit and juices. You can lower your triglyceride level with diet, exercise, and a high fiber diet.

Trans Fats:Margarine is the largest source of Trans Fatty Acids, although they are also found in shortenings and in the partially hydrogenated oils that are used in baked goods and fried foods. The partially hydrogenated oils stay solid at room temperature and don't go rancid as quickly. These fats are now thought to be dangerous to your health.

GOOD HEALTH IS THE GREATEST GIFT YOU CAN GIVE YOUR CHILD.

In this complete package Jay Gordon, M. D. has assembled his 15 years of practical knowledge into an easy-to-use, children and family health program in 3 books, 6 audios and 2 videos.

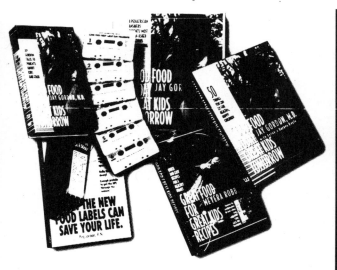

GOOD FOOD TODAY, GREAT KIDS TOMORROW

An easy-to-read, user friendly practical program for parents, grandparents and other childhood care providers. It answers the most often-asked questions about making correct food choices for happy, healthy children.

Written and recorded in an informal and personal style, pediatrician/nutritionist Gordon clearly explains the power of diet for a child's health and well-being. Light-hearted illustrations, discussions and interviews are coupled with precise recommendations which give parents simple changes they can make in their child's diet—changes that will have life-long beneficial results.

- Solving Your Child's Weight Problems.
- Myths About Food
- The Foods Your Child Really Needs
- Delicious & Nutritious Meals, Snacks and Lunch Box Delights
- Special Time Eating—Grandma's House, Fast Food Restaurants, etc.
- How to Eliminate Dangerous Junk Foods.
- Saying "Goodbye" to Diet-Related Diseases.
- Overcoming Food Allergies, Hyperactivity, Childhood Illnesses, Flus and more.
- Eliminating Bulimia and Anorexia.
- How to Talk to Your Kids About Food that Really Works.
- A 14-Day Transition Plan to a Healthier Family Diet.

BOOKS

GOOD FOOD TODAY, GREAT KIDS TOMORROW
by **Jay Gordon, M. D.** with **Antonia Barnes Boyle.**
The easy-to-read, practical book for parents which answers the most often-asked questions about making correct food choices for happy, healthy children. Pediatrician/nutritionist Gordon clearly explains the power of diet for a child's health and well being. *232 pages.*

GREAT FOOD FOR GREAT KIDS RECIPES:
Quick and Easy Recipes for a Healthy Family.
by **Meyera Robbins** whose healthy and delicious meals were an instant *hit* in her Los Angeles restaurant. With new and exciting meals springing from her kitchen at home, Meyera is a *hit* with her daughter Simone and her husband Jay Gordon on a daily basis. Learn how to cook healthy kid-tested foods that taste great! Over **200 easy-to-follow recipes** that make preparing and eating healthy meals a wonderful experience for the whole family. Learn how to shop for healthy foods, and create delicious meals with no sugar, fat, or salt. *200 pages.*

HOW THE NEW FOOD LABELS CAN SAVE YOUR LIFE!
by **Peg Jordan, R. N.,** journalist, and consumer health advocate. This eye-opening book presents fresh insights on how to read the new food labels to make healthy food choices, prevent chronic, life-threatening diseases and achieve optimum health. *144 pages.*

AUDIOTAPES

GOOD FOOD TODAY, GREAT KIDS TOMORROW: In this insightful six-volume audio set, Dr. Jay Gordon answers the most often-asked questions about making correct food choices for healthy, happy children. Covering birth to adolescence, you'll learn how to set healthy eating patterns today that will lead your children to a lifetime of smart choices. The tapes cover how to handle school lunches, the challenges of special times such as parties, holidays, and vacations, the problems of obesity and eating disorders, and a host of other timely topics that concern every parent. *6 audiotapes.*

VIDEOS

GOOD FOOD TODAY, GREAT KIDS TOMORROW: Join Dr. Jay Gordon and other parents in a lively round table discussion that will improve the way you and your family eat – forever! This video covers tough subjects such as junk food cravings, healthy meals and snacks, school lunches, self-esteem, peer pressure, and much more. Approx. *One Hour.*

JAY GORDON TALKS TO KIDS ABOUT FOOD: Entertaining one-on-one talks with some of America's most health conscious kids. Contains information for all children's age groups. Learn new and exciting ways to help your children begin eating right – today! You'll be giving your kids the gift of good health! Dr. Jay Gordon's unique approach will teach you how to motivate your children to develop healthy eating habits that will last a lifetime. Watch this program with your whole family! It's packed with ideas that ensure better health. Approx. *One Hour.*

O R D E R   F O R M

Send To: **Michael Wiese Productions**
11288 Ventura Blvd., Suite 821, Studio City, CA 91604

Please send me the following:

Quantity		Price	Sub-total
____ **THE COMPLETE SET** (Regular Price $125.70, SAVE $15.75!!) You receive all the following six items.		**$109.95**	_____

Or you may order each item individually:

	Price	Sub-total
____ GOOD FOOD TODAY, GREAT KIDS TOMORROW *book*	**$17.95**	_____
____ GOOD FOOD FOR GREAT KIDS RECIPES *book*	17.95	_____
____ HOW THE NEW FOOD LABELS CAN SAVE YOUR LIFE *book*	9.95	_____
____ GOOD FOOD TODAY, GREAT KIDS TOMORROW *audio set (6)*	39.95	_____
____ GOOD FOOD TODAY, GREAT KIDS TOMORROW *video #1*	19.95	_____
____ JAY TALKS TO *KIDS* ABOUT FOOD *video #2*	19.95	_____
Sub-total		_____

Shipping & Handling $4 per item or $12 for the complete set.	

SHIPPING/HANDLING (see left) _____
CA Residents add 8.25% **SALES TAX** _____
TOTAL ENCLOSED $ _____

Please make check payable to Great Kids Partners. Please allow 3–4 weeks for delivery.

CREDIT CARD ORDERS CALL
1-800-379-8808

❏ Master Card   ❏ Visa

Credit Card Number:

_____ • _____ • _____

Expir. Date:_____

Cardholder Name:

Cardholder Signature:

NAME:

ADDRESS:

CITY:

STATE: _____ ZIP _____

TELEPHONE: